Controlling Herpes Naturally

A Holistic Approach to Prevention and Treat~~ment~~

Michele Picozzi

Controlling Herpes Naturally: A Holistic Approach to
Prevention and Treatment

Copyright © 1998 by Michele Picozzi

Credits for specific material reprinted appear on pages 71-73.

Published by
Southpaw Press
1653 S. 2500 E.
New Harmony, UT 84757
www.herpesnomore.southpawpress.com

Cover design and page layout by Robert Henslin.
Printed in the United States of America on recycled paper.

First printing, 1998
Second printing, 1998

Library of Congress Catalog Number: 97-68478

ISBN: 0-9658600-0-0

"The best doctors in the world are Doctor Diet, Doctor Quiet and Doctor Merryman."

—*Jonathan Swift*
(1667–1745)

C O N T E N T S

CONTENTS

ACKNOWLEDGMENTS

This book would not be possible without the support, kindness and generously-given resources of others. I gratefully acknowlege each of their contributions, and also

- ❧ To my husband for his unwavering support and for making this writing life possible.

- ❧ To Rob and Michele Henslin for their early and on-going support and for seeing the possibilities.

- ❧ To Joni Loughran and Paula Kout for their contributions that provided special and important details and to Jonni McCoy for emotional and editorial support.

- ❧ And to Rob for his infinite patience, sense of humor, and incomparable design skills.

INTRODUCTION

The herpes simplex virus (HSV) has outwitted man and medicine for centuries. It is a formidable foe as it exerts a tenacious and permanent hold deep within in the human body. After an initial episode some individuals never see herpesvirus surface on their skin again; others have occasional bouts while others persevere with chronic outbreaks. While not an inherently fatal condition, herpesvirus outbreaks in the average, healthy individual are inconvenient, uncomfortable, and at times embarrassing because of the sometimes intimate nature of the condition.

This book is intended to fill a gap in information and self-care in dealing successfully with herpesvirus since traditional or conventional medicine offers people with herpes very few treatment options. At present, there are only a couple of prescription medications for use under certain conditions that offer mostly short term relief. More drug treatments appear to be on the horizon, but as yet there is no word on their release, effectiveness, or possible side effects. On the other hand, there are many remedies available now to *people with herpes* (which hereafter will be referred to as PWH and PWGH for *people with genital herpes*) that are inexpensive, easily obtained, and offer both short- and long-term solutions.

Primarily, they involve diet and lifestyle changes, vitamins, herbs and even exercise to relieve herpesvirus symptoms. In many instances, they may keep the virus at bay by coaxing the body to return to a healthy, balanced state through a newly strengthened immune system.

Immunity is at the heart of recurrent herpesvirus. For many, the quality of immune function forms a direct link between the frequency, duration, and severity of herpesvirus outbreaks, regardless of where they occur on the body. Diet, lifestyle, stress all have a big impact on how well or how poorly your immune system functions. Eating highly processed foods, too many sugary foods or foods high in the amino acid arginine all lower resistance to herpesvirus and court its return. An immune system depleted by continuous emotional or physical stress, also sets the stage for herpesvirus outbreaks. Ultimately, the strength of your immune system is determined by what you eat and how you live your life.

In large part, the book is the result of my education in treating my own oral herpes, caught during early childhood. The fair skin and overly sensitive nervous system I inherited combined with the poor eating habits in my teens and twenties and later a chronically stress-filled life invariably increased my risk of frequent outbreaks. My interest in alternative remedies and my strong desire to not to suffer propelled me to search for solutions. Later, I noticed there was a pattern to my outbreaks. Further investigation showed that the circumstances surrounding them were mostly in my control. I then decided to pay closer attention to how I dealt with stressful situations (especially the ones I had no control over) as well as what I ate and the vitamins I took. Over time, I discovered what worked for me: A combination of a diet higher in fresh green vegetables, and fewer processed foods and sweets, increasing my daily intake of B complex vitamins, more rest (particularly during busy times) plus a regular hatha yoga and meditation practice. These actions proved key to keeping my herpesvirus in check.

The origins for writing the book have their roots in an article I wrote for *Yoga Journal* which appeared in October 1995. In researching the article, the only books on herpes available to consumers were written in the early 1980s, at the height of the media coverage on the precipitous rise in cases of genital herpes. Many of these books now are out of print or missing from library shelves.

This book's purpose is to serve as a comprehensive self-help guide so you can better understand how herpesvirus works in the body and how you can keep it under control. In the pages ahead, there are many suggestions you can put into practice immediately. There are guidelines for eating well, living better, handling stress, basic hygiene, dealing with sugar cravings, along with recommended dietary supplements, and specific hatha yoga postures that support immune function. However, they all require that you take an active role in balancing your life so the threat of herpesvirus no longer rules your life.Finally, there is a list of resources to help you get well and stay that way. I hope you will find the information useful and helpful in your commitment to better health.

Michele Picozzi
August 1997

Chapter 1

What's the Big Deal?

At a time when attention and research is focused on higher-profile illnesses involving impaired immunity such as HIV/AIDS, lupus, and chronic fatigue syndrome (CFS), there is another ailment that probably causes more human suffering than any other. It hardly receives any media coverage or nearly as many research dollars as other diseases that reflect a state of impaired immunity. Yet it is just as common and infectious as it was before AIDS. The ailment is herpes simplex virus (HSV).

Nearly 15 years has passed since herpes—primarily genital herpes—last created a stir in this country. Back then, knowledge of acquired immune deficiency syndrome was just emerging. Before AIDS became a crisis, genital herpes was the most feared and dreaded sexually transmitted disease (STD). However, millions continue to experience painful recurrences of genital as well as facial herpes.

Herpes has been a curse of mankind since it surfaced more than 2,000 years ago. The virus comes by its name from the ancient Greek word *herpein* meaning "to creep," fitting since diseases in ancient times were classified by their appearance. In 4 B.C., Hippocrates, the father of modern medicine, coined the medical term—*apthous stomatitis*—for the blisters that accompany an outbreak of herpesvirus. Herpes actually is a collection of some 50 viruses. Over the last 30 years, medical science has identified 8 different types of herpes that affect humans. Most people are affected by the most common forms of the herpes simplex virus, HSV-1 and HSV-2, which cause both primary and recurrent infections. HSV-1 is responsible for outbreaks appearing above the waist—although outbreaks can happen anywhere on the body. HSV-2 occurs below the waist.

Despite the back seat herpes has taken in this age of considerably more life-threatening immune-related illnesses, reports from the Centers for Disease Control (CDC) find that approximately 1 in 3 people in the United States has been exposed to the highly contagious herpesvirus. Other studies say that 30 percent to 60 percent of U.S. children under age 10 have been exposed to the virus. Researchers at the University of California at Berkeley have estimated that 60 percent to 90 percent carry HSV-1, most of whom most likely picked up the infection during childhood. In early 1997, the *New England Journal of Medicine* put the figure for Americans with facial herpes at 1 in 5.

Mostly these figures translate to approximately 30 million to 55 million Americans having experienced cold sores, fever blisters, genital blisters, shingles (a painful inflammation of the sensory nerves), chickenpox, infectious mononucleosis (caused by Epstein-Barr virus or HSV-4), or cytomegalovirus (CMV) sometime in their lives.

Genital herpes, which affects about 20 percent of the sexually-active adults in the United States, infects between 200,000 and 400,000 each year, according to a recent report issued by the CDC. An article in *Patient Care* (Feb. 28, 1995), which cited an estimated 30 million cases of genital herpes in the United States, reported that primary care physicians are seeing an increasing number of genital herpes infections. It wasn't always this way. Herpesvirus, as a medical condition of any consequence, was seldom mentioned in medical journals *before* 1966, about the time the sexual revolution took off. According to Stephen Sacks, M.D., the author of *The Truth About Herpes* (Gordon Soules, 1988), the most significant development in the increase of people contracting herpes is the introduction of the birth control pill. He writes, "As we left behind condoms and foam for the convenience of the IUD and the Pill, we left behind these unnatural, but effective barriers to infection."

Historically, genital herpes finds its way most often to whites from 15 to 29 years old, and affects more woman than men. According to Phyllis Stoffman, B.S.N., M.H. Sc., and author of *The Family Guide to Preventing and Treating 100 Infectious Illnesses* (John Wiley & Sons, 1995), most people will have a recurrence within six months of their first episode. By contrast, shingles will affect only 10 percent to 20 percent of the population, but the risk increases past age 50. One over-the-counter drug manufacturer has put the infection rate in the United States for oral and facial herpes recently between 60 percent and 90 percent of the population, most over age 50, with anywhere from 20 percent to 40 percent experiencing recurring outbreaks.

While the statistics mentioned here are only approximations of the actual number of people with herpesvirus (PWH) and apply only to the United States, HSV-1 and HSV-2 are common throughout the world. The high numbers of exposure and recurrences also reflect the insidiousness and remarkable staying power of herpes. Once contracted, HSV-1 (usually through the mouth from kissing or sharing the same utensils or towels) or HSV-2 (typically through the genitals or anus through sexual contact), herpesvirus *never* leaves the body. After infection has occurred, herpesvirus finds its way to groups of nerve endings, called ganglia, located deep within the body, usually either at the base of the spinal cord or skull. Herpesvirus also can infect the fingers, eyes, and brain, often with more serious health consequences. As yet, there is no prescription drug or over-the-counter medicine that prevents or cures any form of herpesvirus. However, there are a number of natural healing agents that when combined with lifestyle changes dramatically increase the chances of controlling outbreaks as well as lessening the severity and duration of episodes.

The combined reality of herpesvirus' prevalence in the general population and no known cures demand a proactive approach to the problem. This means doing what's necessary to keep both mind and body strong. It's the only reasonable and sensible alternative to controlling future outbreaks and further spreading the virus.

However, when working with the natural remedies in general and with those described here, patience is required. First, you need to find the right combination of remedies that will work for you. For most PWH this means making changes in diet and lifestyle, taking more or different types of supplements, and getting regular exercise or taking up meditation. Regardless of what is done, natural remedies, while they can be safe and effective, take time to work and align themselves with the body's innate ability to heal itself.

Chapter 2

Understanding Herpes

Herpes is classified in the medical world as a recurrent, highly contagious virus. As viruses go, herpes has earned a reputation for being one of the most persistent and pervasive viruses. And herpesvirus doesn't discriminate: It affects every animal species in nearly every part of the world.

Generally speaking, viruses are considered by their very nature to be parasitic because they invade the host and then proceed to set up housekeeping in the host's cellular structure. Since viruses can't survive or duplicate on their own, they instead have the ability to wrap themselves in a protein "shell" to avoid detection by the immune system. In order to multiply, viruses are adept at confusing the immune system by changing their protein markers, shedding their protective protein sheath, and taking up residence in the host's cells. Then they go about their real work: mixing their DNA with the host cell's genetic code. Now the virus can really go to work, spreading through the body unchecked, invading more cells, and wearing down the body's defenses.

Scientists have pegged herpesvirus as one of the most complicated viruses known to man. Some have gone as far as to call herpesvirus the "ultimate parasite." Why hang such a frightening tag on a virus that is most commonly associated with the common cold? The simple explanation is that when herpesvirus has an opportunity to infect, it moves in, hides out in the nervous system and remains with an individual for life. No drug as yet can stop it.

At its core, herpesvirus carries DNA, the basic building block of life. Since herpesvirus lives inside a cell, antibodies that normally would fend off the virus from attack can't get to herpesvirus now inside a cell and destroy it. Part of what makes herpesvirus unique is that it hides in the ganglia (the cluster of nerves that branch out from the spine) or trigeminal ganglion (nerves located in the skull) in the case of facial herpes (HSV-1). Because of where herpesvirus hangs out in the human body, it has proven to be mostly invulnerable to the body's natural defenses. When it sets out to recur, herpesvirus travels down the path of the skin nerves, where it will wage war on skin cells to produce a new set of virus particles. If not stopped, painful ulcers or blisters surface on the skin. Because of the way herpesvirus behaves, it is considered a nerve-infecting virus and skin-blistering disease.

To devise an effective treatment to kill herpesvirus, scientists must devise a treatment that kills off the virus but not its host environment, human beings. Since there are so many viruses that plague humans, medical and pharmaceutical research tends to concentrate its efforts on developing antiviral drugs that will disable whole classes of viruses instead of one or two. Acyclovir, the only prescription drug treatment currently available for treating herpesvirus, works by keeping herpesvirus from duplicating itself. (Chapter 4 discusses acyclovir and the latest drugs and vaccines for herpesvirus now under research in more detail.)

By contrast, the *Journal of the American Medical Association* (Oct. 7, 1992) has reported that childhood herpes may actually lower an adult's risk of getting genital herpes and even AIDS. Some homeopathic doctors have even said that childhood infections may be important in challenging the immune system. They theorize that viruses such as herpes serve to provoke and exercise the immune system, which they say may be essential for vitality and disease prevention.

Common Types of Herpesvirus

While herpesvirus has been around for a very long time, understanding of it has been slow in coming. It wasn't until the '60s that medical researchers were able to identify and then label HSV-1 and HSV-2.

Herpesvirus encompasses about 50 different types of the virus, which all tend to look the same when placed under a high-powered microscope. The common denominator this family of herpesviruses is their uncanny ability to remain in a dormant state until reactivated by some triggering event.

So far, medical science has isolated and identified 8 kinds of herpesvirus that affect people in any significant way. Herpes simplex virus type 1 (HSV-1 or facial herpes, affecting the lips or face) and herpes simplex virus type 2 (HSV-2 or genital herpes, affecting the penis, anus, vagina, buttocks, and thighs) are the most well-known and most frequently contracted forms. However, there is some debate in the medical community on whether HSV-1 and HSV-2 are one virus or two different viruses. The majority of research indicates that they each represent a different strain, but are somehow related. Others say that the herpesvirus that causes genital herpes may be the same one that causes facial herpes but behaves differently on another part of the body. The common element of both these strains is they are extremely contagious, spread by direct contact with the sores or the fluid they contain.

Varicella zoster, (which causes chickenpox and its recurrent form, shingles), Epstein-Barr virus (identified as causing mononucleosis—"mono" or the "kissing disease"—and sometimes identified as the underlying cause of chronic fatigue syndrome), and cytomegalovirus (also associated with mononucleosis and more recently suspected in hepatitis) are classified as HSV-3, HSV-4, and HSV-5, respectively.

Discovered in 1986 by National Cancer Institute researchers, Epstein-Barr virus (EBV) is considered a latent virus, hiding in the body's B cells, and one that can reappear repeatedly. Two years later, another herpesvirus, labeled HBLV, which infects the cells in the body that manufacture virus antibodies, also was implicated in causing the fatigue that accompanies chronic fatigue syndrome. The recently discovered HSV-6 and HSV-7 have been found in people with chronic fatigue syndrome, while Type 6 has been observed in the T-cells of people who happen to have a variety of illnesses affecting their immune systems. In 1994, HSV-8 was first isolated from the lesions of Kaposi's sarcoma, a disease common in homosexual men with AIDS.

The two types of herpes simplex virus that infect most people are HSV-1, which is responsible for outbreaks appearing above the waist. HSV-1 reveals itself on the body as cold sores or fever blisters on the lips or on areas of the face around the mouth and nose. There also is evidence that outbreaks of HSV-1 can happen anywhere on the body.

Genital herpes, caused predominantly by HSV-2, appears below the waist. Currently it is one of the most common sexually transmitted diseases, affecting millions of people in the United States. According to researchers, HSV-2 outbreaks seem to occur more frequently than HSV-1, particularly if the initial infection with the virus was a prolonged one. Men are thought to have 20 percent more recurrences than women, although the reason for this is unknown.

The only good news about this unusually cruel and persistent virus is that the different types of herpes do not cause the same symptoms. Also, being infected with one type does not make infection with the others more likely. However, having one form of herpes does not exclude the possibility of contracting another type of the virus.

Herpes Connection to Other Diseases

Scientists now believe that viruses, including herpes, are linked to illnesses that target the nervous, endocrine, and immune systems. Some recent reports have connected HSV-1 with Alzheimer's disease. Apparently this association applies only to people who also carry the apo E-4 gene. This gene, some researchers believe, is enough to predispose certain people to Alzheimer's.

During the 1980s, evidence of connections between herpesvirus and other widespread illnesses began to accumulate. For instance, as many as 50,000 cases of CMV are contracted in the United States each year, with the 15-to 30-year-old age group the most seriously affected. CMV has the distinction of being least known of herpesviruses that affect humans, and some doctors consider it to be very dangerous. However, 80 percent of Americans over age 40 test positively for CMV antibodies. Research now indicates that CMV, not EBV, causes mononucleosis and is transmitted primarily through sexual contact.

In 1979, the *Archives of Internal Medicine* concluded that HSV represents the great masquerader of our generation. For example, herpesvirus has been implicated in chronic illnesses such as chronic fatigue syndrome, fibromyalgia, post polio syndrome, Lyme disease, lupus, and mild cases of multiple sclerosis.

How to Know When You Have Herpes

Whether it's a first episode or recurring one, you may feel sick or experience some flu-like symptoms before you actually develop any outward signs of herpes infection. Typically, the symptoms that accompany an initial infection are the most severe you'll experience. Unfortunately, the most frequently noted symptoms also mimic flu symptoms or those associated with an upper respiratory infection, and include fever, swollen glands, chills, and fatigue. Eventually, lesions will occur on the mouth, face, or on or around the genitals or anus. It takes the body from 10 to 14 days to react defensively and to mobilize to rein in herpesvirus.

Because the skin around the facial lips is a bit drier than the skin of the genitals, the blisters appear more commonly here. Cold sores and fever blisters typically emerge at the vermilion border of the lip, the point where the thin mucous membrane of the mouth meets facial skin. Before HSV-1 becomes visible and erupts into a full-fledged sore, the affected patch of skin typically will first tingle, itch, then redden and appear puffy. As the blister draws more water to itself, it will grow larger, and often the tiny blisters will run together. Then the painful blister or blisters will fill with a clear fluid or sometimes pus that will ooze and crust over and then vanish in about 7 to 10 days, leaving a darkened patch of skin that eventually disappears as well. Herpes sores that continually weep with pus should be examined by a medical professional and treated accordingly.

From the time the skin tingles or itches until the sores or blisters are completely healed, PWH should treat the situation as a highly contagious one, and take whatever precautions necessary so as not to infect others.

Skin that is overly moist or whose natural protection has been compromised by injury or trauma is an ideal setting for herpes transmission, since the virus enters the body through microscopic breaks or tears in the mucous membranes. This means most areas of the body are likely territory for herpesvirus outbreaks. While the initial infecting bout with HSV-1 and HSV-2 frequently lasts longer and is considered more severe and painful, subsequent outbreaks that follow one after another can be equally painful.

For a certain diagnosis, an examination by a medical doctor is advised. The characteristics of herpesvirus outbreaks are unique, and typically a visual examination of the affected area will confirm infection, as both HSV-1 and HSV-2 are considered external diseases of the skin. However, genital herpes can be mistaken for syphilis or other diseases. In women, HSV-2 can settle on the cervix and therefore go undetected. There are several methods of laboratory testing including the staining of a smear, tissue culture, or blood test for antibodies. The specific blood test for diagnosing herpes is called the Western blot test. However, some medical doctors consider a culture of the blisters or lesions as the benchmark for diagnosing HSV. In confirming genital herpes, polymerase chain reaction (PCR) tests can be up to eight times more sensitive in detecting an infection.

For an accurate confirmation on the type of HSV contracted, particularly with an initial infection, testing is suggested. Dermatologists, medical doctors who specialize in diseases of the skin, are considered the trained medical experts who treat people with herpesvirus outbreaks, although family doctors or general practitioners are qualified to diagnose and treat HSV-1 and HSV-2.

How Herpesvirus Works in the Body

Medical science considers herpes a "slow virus." This class of viruses is characterized by long incubation periods, and is suspected as the cause of persistent and often neurologically-based diseases, that are thought to occur long after the virus' initial contact. After emerging from deep within the body, herpesvirus travels from one cell to another without ever leaving the cellular environment. The virus within the cell fuses with a neighboring cell by persuading it to build a series of bridges. Eventually a giant cell is created. The antibodies already circulating are sent to halt the spread of herpesvirus, but can't do much to defend against the invading virus since they can't easily get inside the cell to attack the virus. Meanwhile, herpesvirus is busy constructing bridges before its growth has progressed to the stage where the cell bursts open. It then hijacks human cells, instructing them to replicate, destroying healthy cells in the process.

What Triggers Herpesvirus to Return

A variety of theories exists to explain what reactivates the dormant herpesvirus in our bodies, but exactly what causes about one-third of the people who have HSV-1 or HSV-2 to have recurrent outbreaks remains a mystery. But there are certain situations that roust herpesvirus from its dormant state deep within the body's nerve endings and send it on a return trip to the skin's surface.

While theories abound on what causes herpesvirus to reappear repeatedly, it boils down to individual tolerance. What spurs herpesvirus into an active state can be of a physical or psychological nature or both. Emotional stress may be a strong factor for some, but for others it is unrelated. An elevated temperature at the site of the original herpes lesion caused by fever or exposure to UV-B rays (found in both sun and shade) often sets

HSV-1 in motion for many, but not for all. The most commonly identified single triggers include eating nuts (particularly the ordinary peanut) or other foods with a higher percentage of the amino acid arginine (such as chocolate), exposure to sunlight, fever, being physically or emotionally run down (often these go together) or by experiencing chronic anxiety, worry, and even ambivalence. Women with compromised immune systems also have recurrences that are more frequent or last longer or both.

The herpesvirus varicella zoster, which first manifests itself in childhood as chickenpox, recurs in adulthood as shingles. When VZV re-emerges later in life, it typically is attributed to chronic stress, aging, or impaired immune function. Opinion, however, varies on whether HSV-1 or HSV-2 has the highest incidence of recurrence. Again, subsequent outbreaks may depend on the individual, their general state of health, and exposure to things and situations that can trigger an outbreak. While the debate goes on about rate of return, the general con-sensus among health professionals is that the immune system must function well and physical and mental stresses be kept at a manageable level if herpes is to be kept under control.

The following are the most common situations that have been found to trigger a herpesvirus outbreak:

- **Foods high in arginine.** Peanuts, sunflower seeds, chocolate, soybeans, gelatin, carob and coconut are high in arginine content. Almond paste, a common and often hidden ingredient in many baked goods, also can trigger a negative reaction in sensitive individuals. Onions, raw or fried, also should be avoided.
- **Ultraviolet light.** UV-B has been isolated as a trigger of facial herpes. Exposure to sunlight, particularly where and when rays are the strongest—beaches, mountains, lakes, and between 10 a.m. and 2 p.m.—should be avoided.

PWH should use a sunscreen of SPF-15 or higher and wear a hat with a brim that covers the face. UV-B also has been linked to certain types of skin cancer.

- **Using known immunosuppressants.** Cigarettes, alcohol, recreational drugs, and sugar all have been proven to suppress immune-system function. Chronic or excessive consumption of these substances puts PWH at a distinct disadvantage at keeping herpes outbreaks at bay.
- **Increased internal acidity.** This can occur when stress levels are elevated or from eating foods that contribute to an over-acidic condition in the body. The most common offenders in this category are sugar, white bread, and other highly-refined foods.
- **Menstruation.** While not conclusively proven because the pattern of recurrence can be intermittent, some women are more vulnerable to outbreaks before the start of their periods because of the significant hormonal changes taking place.
- **Strenuous physical activity.** This can tax the body's resources, depending on current physical condition and stamina level. More studies though are finding a distinct link between suppressed immunity and intense periods of exercise.
- **Trauma to the skin.** Recurrences are known to appear at the site of an injury, and routine dental procedures can trigger outbreaks for some PWH.
- **Increased moisture or friction.** Both conditions are present during sexual intercourse.
- **Seasonal changes.** Those with oral or facial outbreaks are especially vulnerable when the body transitions from spring to summer and summer to fall. Traditional Chinese Medicine maintains that certain bodily organs undergo a

period of change during seasonal transitions. For example, in the spring the liver is under stress and during the transition from summer to fall the lungs are vulnerable.

(**Illness or disease.** With the immune system fighting off other predators, it can become taxed, giving the latent herpesvirus an opportunity to reappear. It should come as no surprise that the common cold is one of the most precipitating factors to an outbreak of facial herpes.

(**Stress, stress, and more stress.** Several theories that suggest that psychological stress by itself can arouse the dormant herpesvirus. The #1 factor responsible for repeated and frequent outbreaks is stress, writes Dr. Richard Hamilton in *The Herpes Book* (J.P. Tarcher, 1980), citing experience with hundreds of PWH. Emotional stress does two things to the body: it can suppress the body's natural antiviral agent interferon and also hinder the body's ability to make the antibodies it needs to fight any type of infection. How psychological stress affects PWH will be discussed in more detail in the next chapter.

How Herpes Communicates with the Body

As decidedly invasive and persistent as herpesvirus is, it does have its own way in communicating with our bodies to warn us that the dormant virus is about to reactivate. The medical term for this phenomenon is prodrome, defined as the warning our bodies send to our brains to signal an impending attack before the main set of symptoms appear. One survey indicated that more than 50 percent of PWH say they experience one or more prodromes, or internal warnings, before an outbreak. These signs and sensations are thought to happen in 90 percent of recurrences and typically occur at the exact site of previous infections. Recognizing these "on-alert" symptoms when they first occur can be a PWH most valuable asset in controlling outbreaks and spreading herpesvirus.

One theory to explain prodromes finds that as herpes viral particles move from the ganglia toward the skin cells, they may irritate the nerves slightly and thereby create the sensations known as prodromes. Another hypothesis supposes that as these affected cells swell, die, and disintegrate, they cause the itching and tingling that serve as warning of an impending herpesvirus outbreak.

Experts agree that skin sensitivity is the most noticeable early warning people with HSV-1 and HSV-2 routinely experience—specifically, tingling, itching, or stinging sensations near the place on the skin where the initial or previous herpesvirus outbreaks occurred. These prodromes can last from a few minutes to hours or even one or two days. Even though PWH experience these warning sensations, the developing lesions for whatever reason are stopped in their tracks, leaving PWH with a much less severe episode to contend with or no outbreak at all.

Prodromes vary from person to person. By becoming aware of the internal signs or signals your body is sending, it is possible to help minimize the length and discomfort sure to come. Equally important, a prodrome signals that it's time to take the necessary precautions to avoid infecting others. Until recently, the point at which herpesvirus can be passed from one person to another was undefined. Recent laboratory tests, however, have demonstrated that contagious virus particles can be shed and transmitted at the outset of warning sensations, before the development of any blisters. In November 1995 *Vogue* reported on research that showed that overwhelming evidence exists that herpesvirus can be spread even when no visible sores are present.

**Since herpesvirus is spread only by direct contact, the
wise, responsible, and kind course of action is to avoid all
close physical contact—kissing, intercourse, sharing towels,
toothbrushes, lipbalm, etc.—at the first sign of any
internal warning sensation.**

The prodromes most often reported by PWH include:

❨ *Crawling*—the sensation that something is crawling or creeping beneath the skin.

❨ *Heat*—a warm throbbing at the site.

❨ *Invisible scratch*—feeling as if there were a slight abrasion on the skin, but none is visible.

❨ *Isolated sensations*—sometimes similar to the tingling or pins-and-needles sensation described later in this list, but restricted to a different and seemingly unrelated part of the body. For instance, one PWGH reported feeling a specific sensation in her foot preceding a herpes outbreak.

❨ *Itchiness*—the feeling that something is on or just below the skin or that a rash is on the verge of appearing.

❨ *Malaise and general fatigue*—the general complaint of feeling "sick and tired" but is nonspecific. That is, no one part of the body feels particularly bad, but simply feeling a general sense of not feeling well.

❨ *Muscular aches and pains*—the muscles near the nerve paths involved in the migration of virus particles sometimes ache or throb with a dull pain. In the case of oral herpes, PWH sometimes report that their cheek and jaw muscles ache.

❨ *Neuralgia*—an impending viral attack is sometimes characterized by pain, usually mild, but sometimes quite sharp, radiating through the lower back or down the legs or throughout the planes of the face.

❨ *Phantom inflamation*—the area feels inflamed, and perhaps is even warm to the touch, yet is not visibly so.

- « *Pins and needles*—as if a small patch of skin had "fallen asleep," much as a limb in a cramped position will lose sensation and then "come back to life."
- « *Pressure*—the sensation that something is pushing under the skin or pressing up against the surface.
- « *Prickly sensations*—like tiny jabs in the skin.
- « *Slight surface achiness*—on or near the site of past outbreaks.
- « *Swollen glands*—lymph glands swell when an infection takes hold and the immune system is stimulated. Although this symptom usually accompanies the primary or initial attack of herpesvirus, many PWH report swollen glands as a prodromal symptom. Perhaps the immune system anticipates the impending viral infection and begins to gear up against it, with increasing activity in the lymph nodes.
- « *Tingling*—an almost ticklish feeling, sometimes as if there were a slight vibration beneath the skin.
- « *Touch sensitivity*—the skin feels sore or as if a pimple were about to erupt.
- « *Twitchiness*—as if there were a slight spasm or twitch beneath the skin.

Prodromes almost always mean that the HSV has been reactivated within the body, whether or not outward physical signs such as blisters appear. Sometimes the course of the recurrence has been short-circuited, but the reasons for this aren't clear. False prodromes, as they are called, are known to occur more frequently in PWH who take regular doses of acyclovir, the most widely prescribed drug for genital and facial herpes.

Chapter 3

Pointers on Prevention

With herpes, an ounce of prevention is worth a pound of cure, and maybe even more for chronic sufferers. Flare-ups, despite the best efforts to prevent them, can occur when least expected. When preventive measures fail, natural remedies can come to the rescue.

The connection of mind and body to recurrent herpes outbreaks is a relatively new theory and one worthy of serious consideration by any PWH who seeks to control future herpesvirus outbreaks. The consensus among alternative and some traditional health practitioners is that stress is the #1 precipitator of recurring herpesvirus outbreaks. Emotional stress is usually cited first, but there are other stressors that should be considered as well.

Coping with Stress

Oscar Gillespie, Ph.D., makes the connection between herpes outbreaks and stress in *Herpes: What to Do When You Have It* (Grosset & Dunlap, 1982). He writes that herpesvirus can become the path of least resistance for the body, since a disease such as herpes can establish a pattern within the body, thus weakening normal recovery processes and immune defense capabilities.

Stress, whether it's good or bad, is normal and a regular part of everybody's life. Too much, though, can stretch our capacity to adapt just so far before detrimental effects occur. The most common example of this is heart disease. The combination of health problems associated with this potentially life-threatening situation are revealed usually by specific physical symptoms that are aggravated by long periods of continued stress and, often by eating foods high in salt and fat.

Chronic stress ratchets the body's nervous and hormonal systems up a notch or two to where its built-in mechanisms for adapting to and coping with stressors begin to fray and eventually break down completely. Consequently, the body's ability to deal with foreign agents or internal changes also is impaired. For PWH, this means prolonged stimulation of the nervous system can easily be channeled into herpesvirus activation at a time when the functions performed by the immune system will be greatly diminished, resulting in more outbreaks of greater duration. This can be treacherous because too often the stress response will occur way beneath our awareness and surface only through physical symptoms such as herpesvirus outbreaks. Gillespie believes it's as if herpes becomes the path of least resistance for the stresses of the world until that connection is broken.

Overdoing It

Often high levels of stress are self-imposed, a direct result of doing too much or feeling overwhelmed. Whether it be work, working out, socializing, or volunteering to solve anothers or the world's problems, any of us can get caught up in them to the extent that health and well-being is put at risk. We live in a speed-crazed world, where racing against the clock is an accepted way of life. American culture rewards us more for moving fast rather than going along at pace more suited to our own natural rhythms.

Learning how to slow down, even when you want to, can feel like an experiment in foolishness or frustration. But recurring bouts of herpesvirus represents a clear signal to PWH that a real effort to slow down the pace of your life should be considered. At the very least, from time to time entertain the notion that there is real value in doing nothing. If not, herpes will win out time and again.

Besides the stress involved in pushing ourselves past our limits, there are other stressors, out of our control, that for some impact the frequency of herpesvirus outbreaks. For instance, some women will have outbreaks only at certain points during the menstrual cycle, but the point in their cycles that trigger outbreaks can vary from woman to woman. One study suggests that more women develop recurrences 5 to 12 days before the start of their next menstrual period than at any other time. Even though birth control pills stop the cycling hormones, they don't seem to diminish future outbreaks in some women of childbearing age.

Other people can become vulnerable when taking certain medications, when they have a fever, or during prolonged and even brief exposure to strong sunlight. Others whose mouths are sensitive may find a session in the dentist's chair can provoke or intensify an outbreak. Direct stress to the skin's surface by exposure to cold, windy, or dry weather conditions, food served at extremely hot temperatures, or biting or chewing lips with your teeth also can leave skin tissue open to an attack.

Getting a Grip

When grappling with the stressful areas of life, it's helpful to understand a few basic principles. First, stress is a subjective state of mind. How an event or situation is perceived often will determine how stressful the mind and body find it. Reactions, the mind experts tell us, are learned behavior. With practice, conditioned behavior and automatic responses can be rethought and eventually reformed.

Stress consultant and author of 11 self-help books Richard Carlson, Ph.D., reminds us to "not sweat the small stuff… because it's all small stuff," which happens to be the title of one of his books. Outlined in 100 brief essays that mirror Buddhist philosophy, Carlson proposes 10 rules of living, based on compassion and patience, to improve the quality of life. His point is that much of our anxiety and inner struggle stem from our busy, overactive minds always needing something to entertain them, something to focus on, always wondering what's next. Just like our bodies, he reminds, our minds need an occasional break from their hectic routine. Instead of trying to raise your tolerance to stress, Carlson suggests lowering it. Excellent advice for living in the over-Information Age.

How do you remain unaffected by events you can't control? Eastern philosophers throughout the ages, recommend practicing detachment—not involving, reacting to or owning another's frustration or anger. It works, but it takes practice. If you can understand and accept that you don't have to respond automatically to what happens to or around you, you put yourself in the enviable position of not indulging in energy-wasting, nonproductive, and ultimately stress-producing activity. There's no denying that life today can be quite stressful, but by acknowledging and anticipating the daily hurdles, you're halfway home in dealing proactively instead of reactively to stress. A good question to ask yourself is, "What's the emergency?" or "What difference will this all make 100 years from now?"

The Overlooked Psychological Connection

Dr. Wayne Diamond, a naturopath and psychotherapist from the Philadelphia area, has spent many years studying the skin condition of his patients. He, like many other health professionals, believes that the skin is a mirror of overall health. "My interest in herpes began," he says, "when I noticed a high number of my patients had forms of chronic viral and bacterial infections." Diamond then undertook a series of clinical research projects that eventually turned up a distinct connection between stress, anxiety, nutrition, and the glandular processes acting in concert to aggravate the skin and goad existing but dormant conditions into action.

According to Diamond, there are two specific emotional states that almost universally precede herpes outbreaks in those who are prone to them. One is internalizing feelings such as anger or fear (anxiety) in times of conflict, and the other is ambivalence or fear of loss. Left unexpressed, these feelings put PWH at risk for recurring infections.

Because anxiety and ambivalence express themselves outwardly in a variety of ways, Diamond has concluded that these particular emotions have an internal effect as well. He maintains that these two mental conditions can effectively diminish the power of the human glandular system which, when so affected, has a tremendous impact on immune function. "When people experience stress and anxiety, their bodies undergo immense changes. Body temperature increases and interferes with how nutrients are absorbed, then large amounts of acid pour into the stomach that then get absorbed into the bloodstream," says Diamond. Overacidic blood can become a very powerful irritant, especially in soft tissue areas where herpesvirus lives. Diamond also theorizes these factors can dramatically increase the chances of a herpesvirus outbreak on the face, sexual organs, or in the instance of herpes zoster, inflamed or irritated tissue anywhere on the body. "If we can understand how stress affects us, we can try to reduce its effects and maintain a healthy mind-connection, " he notes. For PWH, the fulcrum of the balancing act is maintaining a sense of control over your life and sustaining an internal alkaline environment.

Another part of the stress-herpes equation is feeling guilty about your condition. Fretting about the prospect of recurring bouts of herpes only adds to your stress level. When anxious or worried, the mind and body are anticipating or expecting something stressful happening that may or may not occur. While in this state, the nervous system is already engaged and the potential for harm exists.

Frank Fruedberg suggests in *Herpes: A Complete Guide to Relief and Reassurance* (Running Press, 1987) changing the way you think about herpes. Psychologists, he writes, often recommend to patients that they imagine the sores are a result of an allergy. "In a very real way, you are allergic to herpesvirus . . . some people are immune to them, never developing herpes simplex lesions, no matter how often they are exposed, " he explains. Another way to put the situation into perspective is to think in terms of simply having cold sores even though they occur in the genital area.

Reducing Anxiety and Stress

There are many ideas on how to reconsider and reorient the stresses we experiences. Popular author, lecturer, and co-founder of the Mind/Body Clinic at New England's Deaconess Hospital, Joan Bornysenko, Ph.D., reminds us that when our energy is tied up in useless worry and fight-or-flight, we oppose the natural tendency toward growth and wholeness. She finds that meditation is the place where we access the relaxation response and become aware of the attitudes and thought patterns we have that produce stress. Bornysenko calls it "freeing the inner physician."

Here are some other stress-tamers that could work for you:

- *Learn to say no.* With a smile, please—and remember that no explanation of your decision is required. Be firm, polite, pleasant. Practice saying the word. You'll be surprised how well this tactic works in reducing feelings of obligation to do more than you really should.

- *Get at least 8 hours of sleep.* Preferably more if you can. Sleep serves as the physical and mental body's daily tuneup and opportunity for repair. Fatigue from a result of a lack of sleep or anxiety and depression takes your body off course, leaving it open to another round of sores and discomfort. The most beneficial sleep for PWH occurs when bedtime is 10 p.m. or earlier.

- *Meditate.* Substantial evidence exists that meditation supports the immune system by lowering stress, lends a genuine sense of well-being and tranquillity, and helps with negative states of mind as it works on the autonomic nervous system, the part of the body where the fight-or-flight mechanism resides. Start out slowly with 5 minutes in the morning and evening, and add a minute each day until you are meditating for 20-30 minutes daily.

- *Exercise.* Study after study shows that 30 minutes of regular mild aerobic exercise such as walking boosts immunity. However, too much and too long can have the opposite effect. Pace yourself, but get out there and move.

- *Simplify and organize.* Since maintaining your stuff takes time and energy it can be a source of stress. Elaine St. James, who has written three popular books based on her personal experience of unwinding and finding what's important, says there are inner and outer components to the process. The best way to do one or both is slowly over time. St. James recommends one drawer, one closet, or one habit at a time.

- *Avoid high-stress foods.* This includes anything that passes the moderation threshold. Go out of your way to pass on foods that contain proportionately high amounts of sugar and caffeine. Both substances can jangle your nerves and deplete the nutrients your body needs to manage stress. Adding foods high in B vitamins such as brown rice, barley, soybeans, lentils, and chickpeas can help your body cope when anxiety hits. Magnesium supplements also may help.
- *Talk a walk.* When it all becomes too much, opt for an adult time out. Any kind of aerobic exercise (running, swimming, cycling) reduces tension and depression and relaxes muscles.
- *Cry.* The benefits of a good bawl are well documented. Research indicates that tears may remove certain chemicals that have accumulated when we're stressed. Alternative practitioners often encourage their patients to cry often as it cleanses the liver, an essential body organ affected by toxins and unexpressed angry feelings.
- *Listen to music.* A proven anxiety reducer, music can lower blood pressure and help stabilize heart rate.
- *Pet your pet.* Medical research proves time and again that pets are a boon to our mental and physical well-being.
- *Stop. Smile. Take a deep breath.* To keep your mind on an even keel, take a moment every half-hour or hour and stop what you are doing. Smile and indulge yourself in a deep breath, visualizing your worries and problems being carried away with your exhale. Deep, slow breathing automatically calms the mind.
- *Read.* Considered a natural sedative by some medical

experts, it's a cheap and ready escape from daily pressures.

❲ *Take a bath.* Water has been soothing souls and psyches for centuries. A warm to hot bath infused with a few drops of lavender oil and 2 cups of Epsom salts can leave you feeling relaxed and refreshed.

❲ *Stock up on the right nutrients.* Eating right is no guarantee that you're getting all the minerals and vitamins you're body needs. Vitamin expert Earl Mindell has found that the micronutrient content of our daily meals has been reduced dramatically—up to 50 percent—as a result of growing food on burnt-out or overly-treated chemical farm soil. Transportation, storage, preparation, defrosting, and cooking takes away even more. For PWH, to keep the nervous system humming along, daily doses of these proven stress fighters: vitamins B and C, magnesium, zinc, and potassium can be beneficial.

❲ *Put yourself first.* Sound selfish? Not really. When demands on your time and energy climb, taking care of yourself almost automatically takes a back seat. To keep your defenses against stress-related illnesses strong, you must eat right, get enough sleep, take regular exercise, and avoid sugar, alcohol, and cigarettes. How can you be of any real use or service if you deplete your own inner resources?

❲ *Do nothing.* A truly worthwhile pursuit especially for PWH. Really it is. Spending time not doing anything gives your body a chance to turn its energies inward so it can revitalize and restore itself.

❲ *Develop and maintain a strong support network.* Ideally one that's made up of family and friends is important to maintaining well-being and an absolute necessity in times of stress. For PWH, joining a support group or seeking professional help, whether for biofeedback training or counseling to help you cope with having herpesvirus, can provide special support in coping. Check with your HMO, since a growing number of them now offer alternative treatments for stress. More private insurers also are more willing to cover alternative therapies.

The Immune System's Role

If AIDS has pushed HSV-1 and HSV-2 into the background, it has conversely put a spotlight on the workings and importance of the human immune system. The human immune system consists of the lymph nodes, spleen, tonsils, thymus gland, bone marrow, and white blood cells. But it is the thymus gland, a pinkish-gray organ about the size of a walnut located just under the breastbone and above the heart, that provides the body with several important hormones that regulates immune function. The most important of these is the hormone thymosin that regulates white blood cells, specifically T-cells, which fight off bacteria and viruses that cause infections that the body has no antibodies for. Thymosin also enables the T-cells to produce naturally-occurring drugs such as interferon. Biochemist and discoverer of thymosin Allen Goldstein of the George Washington School of Medicine and others call the thymus the master gland of the immune system. The vitamins that support thymus function are the antioxidants vitamins A, C, and E, and zinc, selenium and vitamin B6.

The current state of your immune system is a reflection of your genetic history, the infections you've had, and allergies you've developed, even the vaccinations you've received over the years. The immune system relies on the glandular system to stay strong, and stress can adversely affect both.

One immutable fact about herpes is that the immune system provides the first line of defense against it. Herpesvirus illnesses have been found to be the most common cause of serious infections in people whose immunity has been seriously impaired by AIDS or organ transplant. Research increasingly supports the theory that weak body defenses may be more responsible than the virus itself in activating outbreaks, with stress providing the catalyst in recurring herpesvirus infections.

An immune system that functions at peak efficiency is really your best friend, whether you have herpes or not. It can resist all kinds of infections successfully, ward off allergic reactions, and maintain and repair cells that are constantly changing through growth, decay, or replacement.

Role of Diet and Nutrition

The idea of foods having medicinal or healing value is starting to catch on in the United States. However, and not surprisingly, Traditional Chinese medicine (TCM) and ayurvedic medicine (from India) have worked from this knowledge for centuries. TCM takes the connection a step further by relating food to the balance of a particular organ. "Organs need the taste of food in a certain strength (not too much or too little) to keep their energy maintained," writes Luc deSchepper, M.D., Ph.D., and C.A., in *Peak Immunity* (1989). "Through extensive observation, the Chinese knew exactly which taste relates to which organ. The one belonging to the spleen-pancreas (which the TCM treats as one organ), and important to the immune system, is the sweet taste."

TCM teaches that the body's immune function is dictated by the spleen and pancreas. The spleen also makes white blood cells, the immune system's first line of defense. The spleen is the most important organ in the transformation and transportation of food, says deSchepper. So it follows that if the spleen is not working up to par, then the foods we eat won't be absorbed properly and used to provide energy. If the spleen-pancreas are not working properly, a depressed immune system may be the result.

A condition of "dampness" has an adverse effect on the spleen-pancreas, so raw and cold foods that upset the function of this organ should be avoided by PWH. In addition, raw foods, especially vegetables, are hard to digest. Instead, steam, bake, or stir-fry vegetables before eating them. The nutrients still will be there and your body will be better able to absorb them.

For PWH, diet plays a significant role in reducing or eliminating symptoms. Certain foods such as caffeine, alcohol, and meat (because it is hard to digest), stress the nervous system and should be avoided, particularly when an outbreak is in its early stages. A number of traditional and alternative practitioners also suggest eating lightly, taking plenty of distilled or bottled water and herbal teas, and resting as much as possible.

Besides managing stress, to get herpesvirus under control, it's important to know what to eat and what not to eat in order to keep your body in balance. Wayne Diamond, whose clinical research in viral and bacterial skin infections were mentioned earlier, believes that for the skin to be consistently healthy, good nutrition must be present. He says poor nutritional absorption patterns, along with absorbed toxins, can have a dramatic effect on skin health, resulting in poor skin circulation, reduced skin lubrications and openness to infection.

Beating the Sugar Trap

Sugar is like sunshine: a little can boost your energy and spirits but too much can hurt you. Sugar not only tastes good, but it also causes the brain to release feel-good chemicals such as serotonin and endorphins. We're born with the instinct to seek out sweet stuff, but too often we develop cravings for sugar that follow us into adulthood.

Heavy sugar consumption has been linked to premature aging, several degenerative diseases, cardiovascular disease, liver dysfunction, type II diabetes, osteoporosis, gum disease, weight gain, and impaired immunity. Sugar can weaken the gastrointestinal tract and interfere with food digestion and assimilation. A healthy digestive system is crucial to good immune function. This is important to all of us, but particularly to PWH, because maintaining a healthy immune system is key to keeping herpesvirus from making painful encores.

Author and well-known nutritionist Ann Louise Gittleman calls sweet foods "a devil in disguise." In her book *Get the Sugar Out: 501 Simple Ways to Cut the Sugar Out of Any Diet* (Crown Trade Paperbacks, 1996), Gittleman takes a realistic look at the effects of sugar on the body and offers tips and recipes to eliminate sugar from any type of diet. She and other experts agree that refined sugar acts more like a drug that our bodies need to detoxify than a nutrient-supplying food because our bodies have to use their own mineral reserves just to digest it.

Sugar stalls the immune system by preventing white blood cells from doing their job as germ killers; reduces the body's ability to produce antibodies (the proteins that combine with and deactivate foreign invaders such as viruses); hinders the transport of vitamin C, a nutrient crucial to overall immune function; upsets the balance of crucial minerals such as magnesium and calcium; and neutralizes the effects of EFAs (essential fatty acids), which can make cells more open to invasion by allergens and microorganisms.

Medical studies have found that the immune system's antibody production drops off after as little as 18 grams of sugar—about as much as in a half-can of soda. Besides having no redeeming nutrient value, sugar also interferes with the way the body absorbs B vitamins, a group of vitamins crucial to keeping herpesvirus in check and maintaining a healthy nervous system. The key, as Gittleman points out, is satisfying your sweet tooth without risking your health. Blood sugar equilibrium, she says, is one of the most important but overlooked keys to health. The ideal way for the body to ingest sugar properly is through eating whole foods, particularly complex carbohydrates. The vitamins, minerals, and enzymes in unprocessed foods allow for smooth metabolism of the sugars found in these foods, and then the gradual introduction of these sugars into the bloodstream.

Tips for Reducing Sugar Consumption

⋐ Eat foods that rank between zero and 40 on the Glycemic Index. Foods such as sweet potatoes, slow-cooked oatmeal, grapes, apples, pears, lentils, skim milk, yogurt and soybean bring blood sugar up gradually and contribute to its stability. If you do eat foods that fall in the moderate or high levels (white and brown rice, carrots, applesauce, corn chips, most commercial cold breakfast cereals), try to eat them with some protein to help slow down the body's insulin response. (Books such as Gittleman's *Get the Sugar Out, The Zone* by Barry Sears, and Nancy Appleton's *Lick the Sugar Habit* include the complete Glycemic Index.

⋐ Replace refined sugars with natural sugars such as pure maple syrup, barely malt, rice syrup, fresh fruit, stevia, or FOS (fructooligosaccharides). Avoid honey and fructose. While the body metabolizes these sugars better, sugar is sugar to the body, period. The goal here is to eat less sugar, not to find a steady, less harmful substitute.

⋐ Aim to keep daily sugar consumption under 40 grams, and between 20 and 40 grams if you have regular herpesvirus recurrences. A teaspoon of refined white sugar contains 4 grams of sugar.

℃ If you crave sugar, try eating 4 to 5 small protein-packed meals daily. This will give your blood sugar a fighting chance to even out and eventually sweets will be less tempting. Often, sugar cravings subside by adding more protein to your diet.

℃ Snack on foods high in protein and starch such as hard-boiled eggs, whole grain crackers, soft cheese, fruit and vegetables.

℃ Stay away from fat-free foods. Besides being highly processed, they contain even more sugar to make up for the lack of fat. Also, avoid foods high in carbohydrates such as bread, bagels, and pasta that are high in simple sugars and contribute to blood sugar imbalance.

℃ Substitute complex carbohydrates for simple ones. The complex variety require longer digestion to be absorbed. Foods especially beneficial for PWH include legumes (lentils, chickpeas, kidney beans) and vegetables such as yams, broccoli, and zucchini. These foods with long sugar chains, like complex carbohydrates, release their sugars into the bloodstream gradually and supply the body with a more consistent, even flow of energy. Consider starting your day with a bowl of slow-cooked oats. Old-fashioned oats have been shown to help regulate blood sugar and have a positive effect on the nervous system.

℃ Eat sweets with whole foods to slow down the sugar's digestion and to cut down on cravings.

℃ After a meal or when the urge for something sweet strikes, wait 15 minutes as the urge usually passes.

℃ Read food labels. The number of sugar grams are listed near the bottom of the carbohydrates section of the Nutrition Facts label. Look for foods that contain 5 grams or less of sugar per serving.

❅ To keep blood sugar constant, aim for a diet that is approximately 40 percent carbohydrates, 30 percent protein, and 30 percent fat.

❅ Go through your pantry and cupboards and toss out candy, cookies, sugary cereals, white bread, rice, and pasta. Throw it or give it all away and promise yourself not to replace it. If you must have the food, make a special trip for it and buy only a small quantity.

❅ Chew on cinnamon sticks or cloves to stem sugar cravings. These spices help balance blood sugar by raising insulin, according to studies conducted at the U.S. Department of Agriculture.

❅ Drink a cup of blueberry leaf tea in the morning and evening. Or 2-3 cups of fenugreek seed tea. To prepare, put 2 teaspoons of fenugreek into a cup of water. Set aside for 5 hours, then boil for one minute and drink.

❅ To help with premenstrual sugar cravings, mix up a batch of raw almonds (soak in water for 2 to 3 hours first), sprinkle 1 or 2 teaspoons of cocoa powder over them, then mix thoroughly with a tablespoon of barely malt syrup. Enjoy.

❅ Enlist the aid of supplements. Regular intake of the glucose tolerance factor (GTF) version of chromium is recommended over chromium picolinate to stabilize blood sugar, particularly if you have been a heavy consumer of sweets, bread, and pasta. Take 200-600 mcg daily. For over-whelming sugar cravings, Ann Louise Gittleman recommends taking 500 mg of the amino acid l-glutamine 3 times daily. The brain converts l-glutamine to glutamic acid, the only source of glucose besides sugar that the brain uses for energy.
The antioxidant alpha liopic acid (ALA) has shown promise in helping diabetics control their blood sugar.

About 50 mg a day should help curb cravings. Also, be sure you're getting enough magnesium, at least 300-500 mg daily; increase intake if cravings (particularly for chocolate) are stronger before menstruation. Other vitamins and minerals important to maintaining blood sugar balance are zinc, manganese, B complex, vitamin C, and pantothenic acid.

❅ Siberian ginseng also curbs sugar cravings and keeps energy levels steady while nourishing the adrenal glands.

If stress triggers sugar binges, supplemental formulas specifically to support adrenal and pancreas functions are recommended. Stress and sugar represent a harmful combination to the adrenal glands, which constantly help your body cope with stress. The adrenal glands are closely associated with function of the kidney and liver, two vital organs that rely on proper nutrition and adequate rest for functioning.

Sugar has been proven to block the absorption or speed up the elimination of B vitamins and nearly all minerals. After you eat sugar, both calcium and magnesium are eliminated from the body when you urinate. According to Gittleman, no matter how much of these minerals you take in food or supplemental form, if you take them with a lot of sugar, you will not be able to absorb them.

The key to maintaining balanced blood sugar is protein and essential fatty acids. While diet experts constantly warn about fat consumption, it is not nearly as critical to good health as keeping your blood sugar in balance.

Foods to Add to Your Diet

As food science makes strides in research, strange and fancy words such as *nutraceuticals* and *phytochemicals* are being bandied about. Both help in the prevention and treatment of illness and diseases. Ruth Winter, author of *A Consumer's Guide to Medicines in Food* (Crown Trade Paperbacks, 1995), notes the immune system is very much influenced by what we eat. Phytochemical, as described in an April 1994 *Newsweek* article, is an umbrella term applied to the array of natural chemical compounds found by the thousands in such whole foods as fruits, vegetables, grains, and legumes. The magazine reported that phytochemicals are substances that give other virus-and cold-fighting vitamins in whole foods a supercharged boost.

Phytochemicals contain some important components, such as:

- ❦ *Sulforaphane:* a tumor-blocking substance found in broccoli, cauliflower, brussels sprouts, and kale.
- ❦ *Allyic Sulfides:* found in garlic and onions. These validate the claim that garlic is an excellent natural preventative for colds, flu, other infectious diseases, and chronic conditions such as stomach cancer.
- ❦ *Flavonoids* (or bioflavonoids): found in green plants, citrus fruits, and berries such as currants. These exponentially boost vitamin C absorption in the body, thereby fortifying the immune system against viruses. They also are thought to block cancer-causing hormones from latching onto a cell. Quercetin, a very powerful flavonoid, is thought to be effective against HSV-1 as well as other viruses.

Garlic

This versatile, talented member of the onion family acts like a broad-spectrum antibiotic, killing bacteria, fungus, yeasts, viruses, and parasites and helps to eliminate toxins in the body. Hippocrates, who gave herpes its modern name, used garlic to treat infected wounds and upper respiratory infections. It also may help to control blood sugar.

To many people's dismay, conventional antibiotics aren't effective against viral infections. Garlic or its constituents, notes writer Paul Berner (*The Healing Power of Garlic*, Prima Press, 1996), will directly kill a variety of viruses including flu, herpes, and CMV. It also stimulates the body's natural defenses against these invaders.

Raw garlic holds more benefit than taking it in pill form, and the purple-skinned variety is considered to possess the most medicinal properties. To get the full benefit of allicin, garlic's most active medicinal property against microbial infections such as herpes, it must be fresh, either chopped or crushed. For best results, eat 2 to 3 raw garlic cloves daily or use that amount or more in soups or salads. The best way to extract allicin from garlic, Berner suggests, is to soak the garlic pieces in a mixture of water and alcohol (try a dry red wine) at room temperature for 3 hours.

Since garlic is a strong herb, side effects are possible, particularly in high doses. Two to three or more bulbs daily can cause stomach and skin irritation, nausea, diarrhea, intestinal gas, headaches, flushed skin, increased sexual desire, and insomnia. Cutting back should reduce symptoms. Any serious harm to the body by eating large quantities of garlic usually doesn't usually occur because the discomfort experienced puts the brakes on overconsumption.

If taking garlic raw is inconvenient or too strong, try Kyolic brand garlic made by Wakunga Pharmaceutical Company in either liquid or capsule form. While it is a less irritating form of garlic, it doesn't have as many of the benefits that raw garlic offers, but research finds there is merit in taking it, particularly as a tonic.

Fresh garlic juice, made with a press, can be applied directly to external herpesvirus lesions.

Foods that Act as Medicine

These foods that have been shown to have antiviral and antibacterial activity, including herpes, cold, and flu viruses:

- ❰ Green tea—also packs a high antioxidant punch
- ❰ Quinoa—a high-protein, gluten-free grain that's rich in lysine and vitamins B and C.
- ❰ Garlic—an all-around helper for PWH.
- ❰ Red marine algae—preliminary laboratory research suggests this type of algae inhibits growth of herpesvirus.
- ❰ Olive leaf extract—there is growing evidence for curtailing the growth of viruses and bacteria. Also shown to help heal herpesvirus lesions as well as lessening fatigue.

Some of the most exciting developments on the research front concerning natural herpes remedies focuses on seaweeds and algaes. A Swiss pharmaceutical company has developed a seaweed-based antiviral cream that works on herpes lesions and preliminary tests at an Israeli medical university and anecdotal reports appear to be promising. Another company, Life Energy Systems, markets a red algae-based product under the name of Intracept Pro to halt the growth of herpesvirus.

Foods to Avoid

The molecules of what you eat are metabolized by your digestive system and in turn absorbed by your cells. Making the right food choices may be the shortest route to controlling herpesvirus outbreaks, since the kinds of foods you eat and don't eat can make the difference in controlling herpesvirus flare-ups. However, for changes in fundamental living habits such as diet to succeed, you have to be ready and willing to make and stick to them. Look at it this way: If you're sick of being sick, then giving up the occasional "goodie" won't seem like such a big deal. The tradeoff is exchanging a momentary pleasure for the long-term gain of missing out on the pain and suffering of a herpes flare-up. Another word for it is discipline.

According to Richard S. Griffith, M.D., professor emeritus of medicine at Indiana University School of Medicine and infectious disease specialist, if you feed herpesvirus enough of the right stuff, it may grow furiously, prodding the body to make cold sores, genital blisters, and other symptoms. The alternative is to starve the virus, subduing it so it can't cause much trouble.

The right stuff in the case of herpesvirus is the amino acid lysine, which has been found in clinical and laboratory tests to stifle the growth of herpesvirus. On the other hand, arginine, another amino acid, has been found to encourage the growth of the herpesvirus. One theory is that lysine wraps a protective coat around the cell, barring the virus from penetrating it and taking out the cell's vital components. Griffith believes it is the balance of power, not just the amount, between the two amino acids that determines whether the virus takes over cells and flourishes in the body.

The following foods have high ratios of arginine to lysine and tend to stimulate growth of the herpesvirus.

Foods High in Arginine

- Chocolate
- Nuts, especially peanuts, brazil nuts, cashews, hazelnuts, pecans, walnuts, almonds, and sunflower seeds
- Gelatin (Jell-O®), even the kind sold in health food stores

During times of physical or emotional stress, PWH also should cut down on or eliminate these potentially troublesome foods:

- Coconut

- Popcorn
- Barley
- Corn
- Oats
- Wheat
- White bread, white pasta, and white rice
- Brussels sprouts

Nuts, particularly peanuts because they are high in the amino acid arginine, have gained a notorious reputation for causing herpesvirus outbreaks in many but not all PWH. A negative reaction to nuts is highly individual. If you're not sure if nuts are a primary cause of your outbreak, Griffith suggests experimenting by eating a small amount of peanuts, about 3 ounces or so, before going to bed. If you react, you'll know the very next morning.

Holistic herpes health care pioneer Wayne Diamond also strongly endorses a proactive dietary stance against herpesvirus. He makes the point that since your skin is your first line of defense or barrier against germs, viruses, and bacteria, a healthy mucous membrane is probably your body's second-best defense to blocking the transmission of herpesvirus. To keep skin healthy and strong, he says, PWH must minimize foods that promote acidity or place strain on your digestive system, such as commercial red meat, white flour, and gluten. Also avoid sugar, chocolate, and tomatoes, foods that often trigger allergies. The vitamins important to keeping mucous membranes healthy and strong include vitamin A and beta-carotene, vitamin C with bioflavonoids, and water-soluble B vitamins.

Diamond further recommends staying away from high-acid foods, including sugar, white flour, MSG, fried foods, red meat, nightshade vegetables (tomatoes, eggplant, green peppers, and white potatoes), citrus, hard cheeses, black tea, and coffee. Dairy products and vinegar should be consumed only in small amounts.

To promote alkalinity, Diamond advocates a diet with plenty of green vegetables (but skip head or iceberg lettuce as it has no nutritional value), whole grains, brown rice, pasta (replace red sauce with white or pesto sauce), yams, salads (garnished with a small amount of dressing), and noncitrus fruits. As proteins, fish and fowl are excellent, particularly good in colder weather. Top selections for vegetable proteins include beans, tofu, and tempeh. Avoiding foods high in the amino acid arginine—nuts, peanuts, seeds, excessive cereal grains, and chocolate. The dietary guidelines suggested by Diamond apply to all forms of herpesvirus and, he says, are equally beneficial to other chronic viral and bacterial skin conditions such as eczema, psoriasis, and acne.

Acid-Producing Foods to Minimize or Avoid

Foods that foster an acid state seem to encourage the activation of herpesvirus. Conversely, alkaline-producing foods (such as steamed leafy green vegetables) produce an internal state that discourages herpesvirus from its dormancy.

- Coffee (including decaf); and during outbreaks drink black tea sparingly
- White bread and baked goods (pastries, cookies, bagels, muffins, scones, and croissants)
- Fried foods
- Pizza
- Anything with high fructose corn syrup or sugar
- Processed lunch meats, spreads, and processed cheese
- Conventionally made jellies and jams
- Soft drinks
- Alcohol
- Ketchup and mayonnaise
- Black pepper, excessive salt, and prepared mustard
- White vinegar

- Baking soda
- Aluminum-based baking powder

It's also a good idea to eliminate or cut down on the amount of meat you eat since meat eaters tend to have lower immunity and prone to a variety of chronic and life-threatening illnesses.

Alkaline Producing Foods

For PWH these foods should be consumed on a regular basis:

- Vegetables and herbs
- Fruits (except citrus)
- Legumes (adzuki beans, black-eyed peas, lentils, chickpeas, great northern beans, navy, butter, pinto and kidney beans)
- Whole grains, especially millet
- Seaweeds

Diet Pointers

- Go out of your way to eat fresh, organic foods.
- Vary your diet. Try to eat different foods every day.
- Begin every day with a healthy breakfast.
- Avoid food additives, artificial colors, preservatives, stabilizers, and chemicals such as nitrates BHA and BHT.
- Eat processed foods sparingly. Commercially-prepared ice cream, soda (colas in particular), and candy all fall into this category.
- Stay away from refined carbohydrates and refined sugar. The body must draw on its reserves to break down sugar while using up its supplies of vitamins B1, B2, B6, niacin, magnesium, and others. Also, eating a diet heavy on grains, whole or not, can upset the body's balance and set the

stage for an outbreak.

❧ Focus on eating quality proteins. Foods that contain all of the essential 8 amino acids are called "first-class proteins," and are found in both animal, vegetable, dairy, and seafood products. Your body's requirements for protein depend on the overall condition of your health, current stress level and how well you synthesize the protein you consume. Vary the amounts and kinds of proteins you eat for maximum assimilation. If you are economically and ecologically inclined, mix grains and legumes and other inexpensive forms of proteins.

❧ Juicing is one of the best ways to get your vegetables and increase your intake of beta-carotene and zinc. Especially beneficial to PWH are combinations of beets, carrots, celery, and parsley juices, as they are natural liver cleansers. Add fresh apple, garlic, or ginger for variety.

❧ Shiitake mushrooms have been used by the Chinese for centuries to foster resistance to infection. A compound called lentinan found in the mushrooms has been found to increase immune function by stimulating interferon and T-cell production. Shiitake mushrooms are available in fresh and dry forms.

❧ Try eating edible seaweed. When the virus meets certain edible seaweeds, herpesvirus shrivels and retreats. In experiments conducted in the 1970s on the effect of different kinds of seaweed from the red marine algae family on HSV-1 and HSV-2, spread of virus was reduced by 50 percent and diminished the viability of the pro-herpes activity by 100 percent. One species in particular, Cryptosiphonia woodii, a microalgae found in the inner-tidal pools scattered along the Pacific coast, was found by Scripps Institute to hold back herpesvirus.

❅ Eat only when hungry and only until hunger subsides, not until you are filled to the gills. Push away the plate when you are two-thirds full.

❅ Chew your food slowly and completely.

❅ Pause and be grateful for what you already have.

Both clinical research and anecdotal evidence have shown repeatedly that diet is the most effective in preventing recurrences of herpes outbreaks or in thwarting herpesvirus symptoms in their initial stages. The quicker you move to cut out aggravating foods, the more likely you are to benefit.

Vitamins, Minerals, Amino Acids, and Herbs

Earl Mindell, R.Ph., Ph.D., author of the *Vitamin Bible* (Warner Books, 1985), defines vitamins as organic substances necessary for life in all its forms—growth, metabolism, and physical and mental health. Vitamins are essential to the normal functioning of our bodies and, with few exceptions, cannot be synthesized or manufactured by our bodies. In their natural state, they are found only in minute quantities in all organic food, so to head off deficiencies or to supplement what our diets don't normally supply, it's particularly important for PWH to take supplements. There are 13 organic substances called vitamins and 18-plus elements known as minerals and 8 amino acids that have been identified for proper body function and maintaining good health. Different vitamins, however, fulfill different needs. Some aid the work of enzymes and others join up with hormones that affect the glands and subsequently other organs. Others have a definite role in cellular and immune functions.

The established allowances for vitamins and minerals set by the U.S. government through the Recommended Dietary Allowance (RDA) are automatically low since they are set to meet the *minimum* amount of a vitamin and mineral required to avoid gross nutritional deficiencies. In fact, Roger Williams, Ph.D., who discovered pantothenic acid some 40 years ago, suggested the idea of "biochemical individuality." He maintained that while we all need the same nutrients, the amount can differ greatly from person to person.

Janet Zand, N.D., O.M.D., L.Ac., and co-founder of McZand Herbal, believes that the fruits and vegetables grown today lack the nutritional potency of produce grown earlier in this century. She says overworked, chemically treated soils and pollutants have resulted in a food supply deficient in the vitamins and minerals necessary to defend against serious and chronic illnesses. Zand also favors tailoring supplement intake and dosage to daily or seasonal need and varying the brands of the most frequently taken supplements.

While there is no consensus on how large dosages should be for PWH to maintain health, some practitioners have made recommendations. You should, however, experiment to determine what's best for your particular health situation. In a report issued in July 1996 by the *Council for Responsible Nutrition News,* the National Institutes of Health said that physically active adults many need increased amounts of some vitamins including B_1 (thiamin), B_2 (riboflavin), and B_6 (pyridoxine). Exercise is believed to burn up more of these three nutrients as these B vitamins are involved in the metabolic reactions that produce energy. In the same report, the antioxidants vitamin C, E, beta-carotene, and selenium were found to be important in repairing the oxidative damage caused by the release of free radicals during exercise. Stress and air pollution also tax our bodies resources, and when ill from a viral or bacterial invasion, the body uses up more vitamins and minerals than normal.

The vitamins and minerals that support a strong, responsive immune system are A, E, C, B_6, selenium, and zinc.

Vitamin A important antioxidant and crucial to immune function; manufactures red blood cells and supports health of skin, mucous membranes, hair, and eyes. Also important for producing lysozyme, an antibacterial enzyme found in sweat, tears, and saliva. (15,000-25,000 I.U.) *Sources:* dairy products and fish oils.

Beta-carotene is a precursor to vitamin A and converts into the vitamin as the body needs it. Although vitamin A can cause toxicity when high dosages are consumed, beta-carotene has no such restrictions, as the body uses only what it needs. It also increases the action of interferon, which the body uses to stop viruses from multiplying, and the action of white blood cells against viruses. In addition, recent research in Germany indicates beta-carotene may protect the skin against UV exposure. (10,000-15,000 I.U.) *Sources:* orange and yellow fruits and vegetables especially apricots, beets, carrots, and broccoli.

B complex as a group, these vitamins protect against disease and infections by supporting immune function. Also useful in repairing tissue, strengthening mucous membrane, helping to build blood, and buffering the body against the effects of stress. Helps the body use sugars, fats, and proteins. Recommended dosage is for a complex formula, as it often works with other nutrients to increase the production of hydrochloric acid, which is necessary for digestion. (50-100 mg, 1-3 times daily) *Sources:* most fruits and vegetables; particularly brewer's yeast, whole grains, liver, and kidney.

In addition to B complex, individual B vitamins can be taken as needed for specific support while under stress.

B_1 *(thiamin):* aids in converting carbohydrates into energy; necessary for a healthy nervous system, good vision, skin, hair, and nails. *Sources:* fortified cereals, meats, cooked oatmeal, and spilt peas.

B_2 *(riboflavin):* helps metabolize protein, sugar, fats, and lipids into energy; supplies oxygen to cells; important for red blood cell growth; used by skin and nails. Easily depleted when under stress. *Sources:* milk, cottage cheese, egg whites, brewer's yeast, broccoli, lamb, chicken, beef, and bread.

B_3 *(niacin):* essential to mental and emotional health; releases energy and stimulates circulation; delivers histamines to the bloodstream; metabolizes food into energy; important for maintaining healthy skin. Reduces tension, fatigue, and insomnia. *Sources:* poultry, lean meat, fish, and peanuts.

B_5 *(pantothenic acid):* important for metabolizing food and producing essential body chemicals; supports formation of antibodies, stimulates adrenal function, maintains digestive tract, and protects against respiratory infections. *Sources:* organ meats, brewer's yeast, bran, sesame seeds, eggs, and soybean.

B_6 *(pyridoxine):* helps synthesize DNA and RNA; used to produce hormones, antibodies, and red blood cells; also aids in the metabolism of fat, protein, and carbohydrates. The body's need for this vitamin is directly connected to protein intake: The more protein consumed, the more B_6 the body needs. *Sources:* bananas, chicken, potatoes, peas, spinach, walnuts, liver, oatmeal, and wheat germ.

B_{12} *(cyanocobalamin):* essential for normal function of all body cells, including brain and nerve cells; increases resistance to infection and is key to formation of red blood cells. *Sources:* clams, oysters, mackerel, sardines, crabs, herring, fish, muscle meats, and dairy products.

Biotin: regulates function of skin, nerves, bone marrow, and reproductive glands; also helps metabolize carbohydrates and protein, folic acid, pantothenic acid, and niacin. *Sources:* egg yolks, liver, brown rice, chicken, brewer's yeast and whole-grain cereals.

Choline: essential to liver function and supports the health of the myelin sheath (nerve covering); and aids in utilization of fat and cholesterol. *Sources:* Whole grains, egg yolks, legumes, cauliflower, lettuce and soy.

Inositol: nourishes the brain; reduces fat in liver. *Sources:* citrus fruits, whole grains, legumes, nuts, and seeds.

Folic acid: central to normal cell growth, production of new red blood cells, and protein metabolism; important to immune function; synthesizes DNA and RNA. *Sources:* liver, brewer's yeast, green leafy vegetables, lentils and black-eyed peas.

Vitamin C (ascorbic acid) a natural antiviral agent that stimulates the immune system to produce interferon and enhances function of white blood cells; assists body in processing essential fatty acids (EFAs). May increase resistance to infection by activating the formation of collagen in the skin and the lining in the body's openings. Also promotes wound healing, strengthens blood vessels and helps the body to absorb iron. (3,000-6,000 mg daily or to bowel tolerance) *Sources:* most fresh fruits and vegetables; especially citrus fruits, rose hips, black currants, and peppers.

Vitamin D general immunity enhancer and aid to healthy skin; important for bones, teeth, body tissue, and cartilage. Valuable to nervous system and heart; aids in blood clotting. (200 I.U.) *Sources:* eggs, milk, fish oils, and sunshine.

Vitamin E greatly influences cellular immunity and helps prolong the life of red blood cells; also its antioxidant function may help in the production of antibodies. (400-800 I.U.) *Sources:* vegetable oils, almonds, sunflower seeds, whole wheat, wheat germ, peaches and prunes.

Minerals and Trace Minerals are vitally important to sustaining health; they work with enzymes that are important to cellular function. Deficiencies lead to increased susceptibility to infectious diseases. *Sources:* whole foods, including dairy products, fish, red meats, fruits, and vegetables.

Calcium helps build bones and keeps them strong; also supports healthy cell membranes. (1,000-1,500 mg daily) *Sources:* milk, cheese, yogurt, tofu, sardines, oysters, dried apricots, broccoli, dry beans, wholewheat bread and fortified cereals.

Chromium regulates how sugar is processed in the body and useful in preventing diabetes and treating hypoglycemia. Also protects against high blood pressure and heart disease. Aging, pregnancy, refined foods and strenous exercise deplete chromium reserves. (100-500 micrograms daily) *Sources:* whole grain cereals, brewer's yeast, meat, cheese and thyme.

Copper helps metabolize vitamin C and iron and promotes energy through supporting production of prostaglandins; necessary to maintain blood, bones, skin, and circulatory system. (1.5-3 mg daily) *Sources:* liver, whole grains, seafood, almonds, and dried legumes.

Iron important to immune function. Deficiency can lead to impaired white blood cell response. (10-15 mg daily) *Sources:* beans, peas, whole wheat, prunes, leafy green vegetables, liver and seafood.

Magnesium helps transmit nerve impulses to muscles; vital in assimilation of EFAs. (200-400 mg daily) *Sources:* almonds and sunflower and sesame seeds.

Manganese essential support to nervous system function and active player in resisting autoimmune illnesses. Activates enzymes necessary to release energy. (2-5 mg daily) *Sources:* tropical fruits, nuts, cereals, egg yolk, and some spices such as cardamom, cloves, ginger, and turmeric.

Molybdenum aids in processing carbohydrates and fats and effective against mercury poisoning. (.075-0.25 mg daily) *Sources:* dark leafy green vegetables, whole grains, and legumes.

Phosphorus can reduce the effects of stress. (800-1,500 mg daily) *Sources:* eggs, fish, grains, meat, poultry, cheese, legumes and milk.

Selenium aids in assimilation of vitamin E and boosts its antioxidant properties and plays an important role in maintaining immunity. Not much is needed by the body, but people with autoimmune diseases have been found to have consistently lower levels of selenium. (50-200 mg daily) *Sources:* fish, kidney, and liver; lesser sources include cereals, poultry, mushrooms, garlic, and asparagus.

Zinc considered the mineral equivalent of vitamin C and probably the most important mineral for maintaining the body's antiviral capabilities. Aids in formation of enzymes; this mineral plays a key role in the body's assimilation of vitamins, particularly B vitamins. It has been found that zinc, when taken with vitamin C, is more effective than taking vitamin C by itself. Necessary for wound healing and maintaining healthy skin. Too much zinc (100 mg taken for 30 days or more) can have the opposite effect on the immune system, depressing it instead of heightening its function. Continued overdosing can lead to heart, cholesterol, and thyroid problems. Its effectiveness is lessened if taken with bran, iodine, and such drugs as tetracycline, cortisone, and diuretics.

Vegetarians in particular should take zinc supplements because of their typically high-fiber diets and because the amount of phytic acid found in plant foods interferes with absorption. Zinc also competes with copper for absorption, so it's best to take both. (15-30 mg) *Sources:* oysters, meat, chicken, lean beef, milk, eggs, fish, pumpkin seeds, lima beans, oatmeal, wheat germ, sesame seeds, and brewer s yeast.

Zinc Lozenges (zinc gluconate) stimulates immune function to fend off viruses and is absorbed quickly by the bloodstream. (One lozenge daily; one every 3 to 4 hours during first sign or first 3 days of an outbreak.)

Essential Supplements for PWH

- *Vitamin C* high doses of vitamin C with bioflavonoids or Ester C (vitamin C bound with calcium carbonate) when the first prodrome surfaces. Take 1,000 mg initially, followed by 500 mg, 3-4 times daily until symptom free.

- *Zinc gluconate lozenge or zinc monoglycerate*—for fighting infection. One lozenge daily; one every 3 to 4 hours at first sign or first 3 days of an outbreak. Also protamine zinc, a protein zinc compound that when injected directly in the sore, heals it quickly, says a Virginia dentist.

- *Lysine* to keep herpesvirus from replicating. Take 500 mg daily on an empty stomach for maintenance; during an outbreak, take 500 mg, 3-5 times daily until lesions heal.

- *Licorice root* immune system and adrenal gland support. Take 30-40 drops of tincture, 2 times daily.

- *B complex* for energy and nervous system support. Take

50-100 mg, 3 times a day.

The Lysine Connection

Lysine has distinguished itself as the prime natural remedy for preventing and treating herpesvirus. Many practitioners, both traditional medical and alternative practitioners, consider this amino acid to be the definitive link to controlling outbreaks. Lysine is one of more than 20 amino acids that make up the body's proteins and it's one of the eight or more essential amino acids. Amino acids (which really aren't acids in the conventional sense) are the raw materials your body needs to grow and repair itself. Since amino acids are life's essential building blocks, they are required by every cell in our bodies. Viruses also need amino acids to reproduce.

A deficiency in lysine has been linked to the fundamental weakness and fatigue associated with many chronic and autoimmune illnesses. Stephen Cooter, Ph.D., author of *Beating Chronic Illness,* writes that known lysine deficiency symptoms, caused in part by a high-arginine diet and without viral complications, resemble the basic weakness and fatigue problems that are common symptoms in many chronic illnesses. He believes that lysine is one possible way of rejuvenating the immune system.

Writer Cameron Stauth, who chronicled his five-year experiences with a worsening case of chronic fatigue syndrome in an article published in *New Age Journal* (October 1994), experimented with taking high doses of lysine taken on an empty stomach. He reported a definite reversal in the severe fatigue and general malaise he had experienced.

Lysine also is necessary in forming antibodies so the immune system can fend off whatever invaders challenge it. Lysine isn't made by the body and only is obtained through protein-rich foods that contain it or by taking supplements.

Interest in lysine as a treatment for herpesvirus started with the discovery of adding lysine to a virus culture medium could inhibit viral growth. Further research found that by varying the ratio of amino acids in human cells, growth patterns of herpesvirus in those cells could be altered. The ratio that changed the most was the relationship of lysine to arginine, another naturally occurring amino acid. When there was more lysine than arginine, viral activity slowed. When there was more arginine than lysine, viral activity increased. In *Amino Acids in Therapy,* Dr. Leon Chaitow concluded that diets rich in lysine or aided by supplementation can thwart the replication of herpesvirus. Dietary choices, he observed, can either encourage or discourage "viral-related disease."

Since a high ratio of lysine to arginine seemed to inhibit growth of herpesvirus as well as interfering with the intestines absorbing lysine, researchers theorized that viral production in PWH might be slowed to the point of decreasing symptoms. Several studies on lysine and herpesvirus conducted over the last 15 years, including one at the UCLA School of Medicine, have produced very encouraging results:

- A study in Denmark concluded that when PWH took a prophylactic daily dose of lysine over a long period of time, it was more effective than taken when the patients experienced prodromal signs of a recurrence.
- In a clinical study conducted at Indiana University, 250 patients with cold sores were given lysine in dosages ranging from 312 to 1,200 mg. Only two showed no improvement, while 248 patients did. The researchers concluded that lysine was a definite positive factor in recovering from an outbreak of HSV. They found that

pain was reduced, lesion spread was halted and healing was speeded up.

❝ Popular alternative practitioner and best-selling author Andrew Weil, M.D., finds lysine to be more effective against oral herpes (HSV-1).

❝ Other reports say that lysine helps other herpes-related diseases including Bell's palsy (a type of facial paralysis) and Meniere's disease (a disorder of the inner ear).

Foods rich in lysine are chicken, turkey, beef, lamb, fish, milk, cheese, beans, mung bean sprouts and brewer's yeast. Foods with inadequate amounts of lysine include most grains such as rice, wheat, oats and millet. Pork, though it has more arginine and lysine, probably should be avoided by PWH who have frequent outbreaks or those with weakened immune systems. This is because pigs are exposed to many viral and fungal infections thought be transmittable to humans.

Lysine also helps build resistance to bacteria and can promote a general feeling of well-being. When taking lysine or other amino acids, it's best to take them on an empty stomach and supplemented with vitamins C and B_6.

However, lysine by itself may not be as effective as a preventive tool. This is the opinion of naturopath and psychologist Wayne Diamond, who created Herpanacine,® a dietary supplement for viral and bacterial skin infections. His research argues that lysine use alone can be inconsistent as a prevention tool, and for some PWH, lysine doesn't work at all.

Good Hygiene

Laboratory studies have shown that herpesvirus is quite sturdy. In 1982, UCLA researchers found that herpesvirus can live on a toilet seat for up to 4 hours, on a medical instrument for up to 18 hours and for as long as 72 hours on gauze. Because herpesvirus is so resilient, diligent adherence to good hygiene habits is one very effective way to control its spread.

While confronted with an active herpesvirus infection, PWH should be especially careful to avoid physical contact with others as well as being equally diligent with themselves. This is important since herpesvirus can be transferred to other body parts by touching an active blister and inadvertently moving active virus particles to take root somewhere else on their bodies, resulting in a new infection with its own independent pattern of recurrence frequency, duration, and severity. To avoid this, during an outbreak, wash your hands as soon as you get up, since touching sores while asleep is common.

To minimize the risk of infection to yourself and others, wash your hands—often and thoroughly with *hot* water and soap for at least 30 seconds—especially after using public facilities and having contact with doorknobs, public telephones, shopping carts, facial tissues, and hand towels used by others.

Avoid sharing towels, toothbrushes, clothing, and eating utensils during an outbreak, and watch where you apply that lip balm or lipstick—keep it away from any sores so you don't infect an otherwise unaffected part of your lip.

At the first sign of infection and if blisters develop, toss your toothbrush and replace it with a fresh one and try to keep your toothbrush from touching the edge of the toothpaste tube to avoid spreading the virus and ending up with multiple lesions. After brushing, soak your toothbrush in baking soda to fight germs and then store your toothbrush upright in a dry place. A bathroom's moist air creates an ideal breeding ground for herpesvirus.

Good hygiene also can help avoid cross-infection. If you

and your partner both have HSV-1, HSV-2, or both, don't make the mistake of thinking you are immune from passing virus particles back and forth to each other during an active period. Since you both may carry a different strain of herpesvirus, it is important that you take precautions or avoid physical contact when you're contagious.

Hatha Yoga

While regular, mild aerobic exercise such as walking often has been proven to be an effective way to strengthen the immune system, hatha yoga takes this process a pleasant step further. Hatha yoga by its very nature is the best example of therapeutic exercise. Certified Iyengar yoga teacher and author Mary Pullig Schatz, M.D., summed up mindful self-care in relation to yoga practice: "Yoga postures are one way of reinforcing the message that all is well, and that normal immune function is appropriate. The body thinks 'I am being so well-fed, well-exercised, and well-rested. Let me be well.'"

Hatha yoga is especially useful in offsetting the effects of stress, and since chronic stress has a powerfully negative effect on the immune system, hatha yoga when practiced regularly helps the body rest and repair itself.

Yoga Postures for Building Immunity and Calming the Nervous System

True to its therapeutic nature, Iyengar-based hatha yoga offers PWH a number of ways to soothe and balance the nervous system. Regular practice of poses or asanas, provides an excellent base of support to any or all prevention efforts suggested here. Valued for their ability to calm, energize, and balance as well as resting the mind and body, these 14 poses are considered part of the restorative category. The series shown here was developed by

B.K.S. Iyengar, world-renowned for his therapeutic approach to hatha yoga, and are practiced throughout the world by people with compromised immune systems.

The majority of these asanas are done with the support of a chair, bolster, or firm blankets. Unless you are an experienced yoga practitioner, do not attempt the handstand or headstand pose without previous instruction by a professional, certified yoga instructor.

While the maximum benefit is obtained by doing the entire series in order, if you are new to yoga, a beginning student, or recovering from any illness, do only as many as you can in sequence and hold the poses for as long as is comfortable. Start slowly, gradually increasing time in the pose as your body permits. Do not exert yourself nor hold any pose where you experience joint pain. Also those with CMV or hypertension should not do handstand or headstand poses.

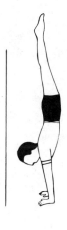

1. Handstand
Keep arms straight. Stretch up vertically. Open armpits. Lift shoulders.

2. Downward Facing Dog
Supported up to 5 minutes. Forehead supported on a block or on a bolster. Weight even on both hands and feet. Legs extend back. Open armpits.

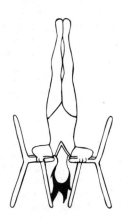

3. Headstand
Supported on chairs. Allow head to hang free. Open shoulders. Stretch up legs.

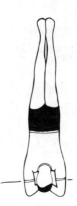

4. Headstand Against The Wall
Folded blanket or sticky mat under head. Keep wrists and hands grounded. Lift shoulders. Extend trunk and legs up. Keep face and eyes relaxed; elbows under shoulders.

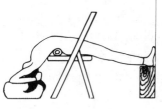

5. Inverted Staff Pose
Support with a chair with head supported on a bolster. Support lower back with rolled up sticky mat or towelFeet supported on block. Hands clasped behind head or extended. Extend legs.

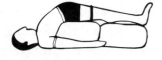

6. Bridge Pose
Use a bolster. Edge of kidneys hit bolster. Belt upper thighs. Feet press against wall. Open chest. Relax throat. Raise feet if back aches.

7. Shoulderstand
Three blankets under shoulders. Belt arms. Extend through legs. Rotate top thighs inward and soften groins. Ground elbows. Relax eyes, neck and throat.

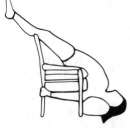
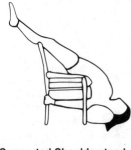

8. Supported Shoulderstand
Blankets or bolster under shoulders. Hands grasp back of chair. Legs against bolster, back of chair or wall. Open chest. Extend legs. Sacrum on chair. Head and neck relaxed.

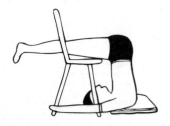

9. Plow Pose Supported
Blankets under shoulders. Thighs supported at least half way on chair seat. Arms extended back along chair legs. Upper back rounds.

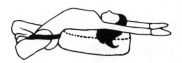

10. Reclining Bound Angle Pose
Belt rests on thighs. Tilt front of sitting bones to floor. Lift pelvic floor. Stretch low back, ribs up towards head. Relax front of body. Relax throat.

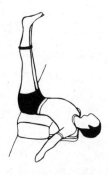

11. Effortless Inverted Pose
Use bolster or two firm blankets folded. Keep groins down. Do not slide away from wall. Feel opening of abdomen and chest. Draw shoulders towards bolster. Rest completely.

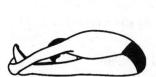

12. Supported Forward Bend
Place forehead on a folded blanket or bolster. Reverse legs after a few minutes.

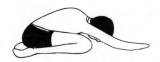

13. Child's Pose
Big toes touching, knees separated to width of chest. Keep buttocks resting on heels. Arms extending, palms on floor. Extend spine.

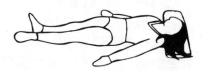

14. Corpse Pose
Place blankets under neck and head. Extend trunk, arms and legs prior to relaxing them. Turn upper arms out, palms up. Quiet mind and breath. Cover front body with blanket if chilly.

Homemade Yogurt Recipe

Yogurt contains essential good bacteria our bodies need. When made without refined sweeteners such as sugar and high fructose corn syrup, it is an especially beneficial food for PWH. Since many commercial yogurts contain sweeteners that prompt adverse reaction in PWH, making your own provides an easy and thrifty solution to store-bought brands.

For the most healthful yogurt, use organic milk and plain yogurt with *live cultures*. To make the first batch, you'll most likely use store-bought yogurt as a starter. A brand with live cultures is essential since the other kind won't work as a starter. For variety, you can use single-flavored yogurts such as lemon or vanilla as starters.

Select a good-size glass jar (16 oz.- 32 oz.) with a screw-top lid. Fill the jar with milk, leaving about 1/2-inch to 1-inch of room at the top. Pour the measured milk into a saucepan. Heat milk over medium heat until it reaches 180 degrees. (A simple clip-on glass candy thermometer works great.) Be sure to keep an eye on the heating milk as it can easily boil over.

Turn off the heat and remove the milk from the stove. Let milk cool until it reaches about 115 degrees. Mix or whisk in about 2 tablespoons of starter yogurt. Pour mixture back into a jar and place lid on tightly. Then wrap the jar in a kitchen towel and hold in place with a rubber band. Place wrapped jar on a heating pad set to low or over the pilot light on a gas stove, and cover jar with a large pot for 5 to 8 hours.

The key to making the yogurt "set" is a correct, constant temperature. Homemade yogurt lasts about 5 days in the refrigerator before turning too tart.

Chapter 4

Pointers on Treatments

What Conventional Medicine Offers

In 1972, approximately six years after the rapid rise in incidences of genital herpes, researchers at the pharmaceutical giant then Burroughs-Wellcome Co. developed the first drug specifically for HSV-2. Clinical trials for the drug known experimentally as BW248-U were conducted from the late 1970s through the early 1980s at the University of Seattle, Emory University, and University of Vermont. The results were encouraging and acyclovir was approved by the FDA for sale as a prescription drug in March 1982 under the brand name Zorivax.

Acyclovir is composed of a synthetic analog of the chemical deoxyguanosine that occurs naturally and is required by cells to produce DNA. It works by subverting the viral genes, not by killing them off but by exchanging live "bullets" with "blanks." Herpesvirus needs a certain enzyme to replicate, and acyclovir fools herpesvirus into using it instead of the proper enzyme. Once herpesvirus accepts the fake enzyme into its genetic structure, the virus can't reproduce itself because technically it is genetically incomplete. As a result, acyclovir acts by stopping replication of the virus and spreading herpesvirus to otherwise healthy cells.

Since acyclovir attacks only the infected cells, it doesn't disturb cells unaffected by herpesvirus. What makes acyclovir so specific in the treatment of herpesvirus is that the particular enzyme it imitates is found only in human cells that have been attacked by herpesvirus.

Acyclovir (Zorivax)—is classified as an antiviral drug and comes in ointment, capsules, liquid, and intravenous form. It is most often prescribed for HSV-1, HSV-2, shingles, and chickenpox. The generic form of the drug became available in early 1997. Existing protocol calls for treatment with acyclovir to begin at the first sign of a lesion, with dosage varying from two doses of 200 mg, 3 times a day or 1 to 5 times a day for 7 consecutive days. However, in severe cases, long-term dosage extends from 1 to 3 years. Maintenance therapy to prevent recurrences typically consists of 2 to 3 daily doses of 200 mg. Current medical literature indicates recurrences of HSV are common after cessation of acyclovir therapy, but with less frequency.

In addition, published studies have shown that acyclovir can't be counted on to prevent either the latent infection state or recurrent infections. Clinical studies have not given any conclusive proof that acyclovir will prevent the virus from moving into the latent or dormant stage even with early use of the drug. In addition, it has no effect on the virus hiding in the nerve ganglia.

Possible side effects of acyclovir include itching or burning of the skin, nausea, headache, dizziness, general weakness, and allergic skin reactions. Side effects of the drug may increase if taken with antibiodics, cyclosporine (an immunosuppressant) and penicillamine, and some cancer drugs. In addition, taking this drug in combination with interferon and methotrexate (used for psoriasis, cancer, and rheumatoid arthritis) may affect the nervous system. Routine use by patients with recurrent genital herpes is not recommended by physicians. Approximately 20 percent of PWH fail to find relief through acyclovir, and some people with AIDS have shown resistance to acyclovir.

Other drugs for HSV-1 and HSV-2 currently being researched or recently approved by the FDA and available by prescription include:

Valtrex (valacyclovir)—is the newest drug treatment for genital herpes offered by Glaxo Wellcome, the manufacturer of Zorivax. It converts to acyclovir in the body. An initial clinical trial of Valtrex indicated that on average healing took nine days, with the accompanying pain persisting for 5 days. In addition, the average amount of time for viral shedding to cease was three days. Although it was found to be well tolerated, the most adverse side effects after taking Valtrex included nausea, diarrhea, and dizziness. Valtrex also is reported requiring 2 doses daily compared with 5 for Zorivax.

Famivir—also is new and specifically treats genital herpes. The drug is made by SmithKline Beecham Pharmaceuticals.

Ribavirin—a synthetic compound that slows the rate of viral replication by inhibiting an enzyme necessary in the production of new viral particles. The drug is under development at ICN Pharmaceuticals of Irvine, Calif. Early tests have shown a reported reduction of pain and new lesion formation in recurrent genital herpes.

Adensoine 5'-Monophosphate (AMP)—is a molecular substance that occurs naturally and is used by cells to synthesize material for a new cell nucleus and assist in cellular metabolism, repair, and replication. Some investigators have found abnormally low levels of AMP in patients with HSV infections.

Isoprinosine (also called Inosiplex)—has antiviral properties and is believed to act against viruses by blocking certain viral processes in infected cells and by enhancing immune factors that are particularly important in fighting herpes.

Bv-ara U—holds potential to be more effective than drugs currently available. Developed by Bristol-Meyers Squibb, it is undergoing clinical trials.

Lithium—a metallic element, it gained notoriety as a treatment for psychiatric disorders. In 1992 doctors at the University of Pennsylvania found that low doses of lithium reduced the severity, duration, and number of recurrent outbreaks of genital herpes.

Other reports of treatment with lithium confirm it has resulted in a reduction in the frequency and severity of genital herpes outbreaks. Ointment containing lithium also has shown promise as an effective treatment for reducing pain and accelerating healing. However, there are side effects such as nausea, vomiting, headaches, disorientation, convulsions, and kidney disease.

Denavir (penciclovir)—the first drug approved for cold sores, was introduced in May 1997. As a topical cream, Denavir was shown in a study that appeared in the Journal of the American Medical Association to provide relief from pain, improved healing by 1 day, appearing to shorten the time the virus was contagious. According to the lead researcher, Spotswood Spruance, M.D., of the University of Utah, people with more severe infections probably experience better results. The most frequently reported side effects reported in the trial were headaches and skin irritation. The manufacturer is SmithKline Beecham.

What Natural Medicine Offers

Herpanacine®

When a trial formula of vitamins, herbs, and amino acids showed positive results on a group patients with recurrent viral and bacterial skin infections, Wayne Diamond, a naturopath and psychologist practicing in suburban Philadelphia, introduced a new formula, marketed under the brand name Herpanacine,® to the public in December 1990. He describes the dietary supplement as a synchronistic formula, stressing the interaction of its 10 ingredients to achieve maximum absorption by the body and provide relief from recurring viral and bacterial infections.

The Herpanacine® formula consists of lysine (to suppress multiplication of herpesvirus); beta-carotene (to cleanse skin layers and the immune system of toxins); L-tyrosine (to balance the nervous system); vitamin E (to purify dermal tissue of toxins and to increase stamina); selenium (to reduce viral cell growth); dandelion root (to reduce excessive acidity in blood and skin and to support liver function); sarsaparilla (to disperse toxins from blood); and astragalus, lingustrum, and echinacea (to reduce viral and bacterial cells in blood and skin layers and to boost immunity).

"I think of it as skin support system from the inside out," says Diamond, explaining that Herpanacine's purpose is to balance the body's overall chemistry, cleanse the skin's layers, build up immunity so the body is able to overcome future outbreaks.

According to literature published by Diamond-Herpanacine Associates, Herpanacine® has a cumulative effect on both the nervous and immune systems. Results typically are seen between the second and sixth months. The longer it is taken, the company advises, the more effective it can be in contributing to overall well-being. Some users also may experience increased energy and stamina.

Suggested uses:

For severe conditions: Take 3 capsules in the morning and 3 more in the afternoon.

For less serious conditions or when improvement occurs: take 2 capsules in the morning; repeat in the afternoon.

For maintenance after condition shows improvement: Take 1 capsule in the morning and 1 in the afternoon.

Note: Herpanacine® should always be taken with food.

Other Fortified Lysine Supplements

Lysine Plus,™ probably the oldest herb-and-vitamin formula for herpes on the market, is made by Quantum. Lysine is the formula's primary ingredient along with garlic, echinacea, vitamin C, propolis, licorice, and goldenseal root. It is available in tablet and extract form, which features shiitake mycelium extract.

Lysine Herbal® by Zand comes in capsule form and contains 500 mg of lysine, magnesium, zinc, vitamin B_{12}, folic acid, and selenium in a base of Chinese and Western herbs that support the immune function.

Helpful Herbs for PWH

‹ **Echinacea** acts as an antibiotic, immune enhancer, and antiseptic, it regulates the glandular system and is a nontoxic way of cleansing the system. Its root extract is believed to show interferon-like activity and antiviral action against the flu, herpes, as well as other viruses. When tincture form is held in the mouth for several minutes, echinacea will produce a numbing effect.

‹ **Goldenseal** performs as a natural antibiodic (sometimes called "Russian penicillin") and antiseptic, it regulates liver function and supports glandular function. Reputed to cleanse and dry the mucous membranes.

‹ **Astragalus** stimulates the immune system and boosts white blood cell levels. Improves resistance to illness. Also restores harmony between kidneys and spleen and supports liver function.

Siberian Ginseng serves as a good overall tonic for increasing energy and enhancing physical and mental well-being. Strengthens the adrenal glands, improves vision, and supports the nervous and cardiovascular system. Boosts resistance to stress and infection.

Licorice acts as an anti-inflammatory and has antiviral properties. Protects the liver and supports adrenal function. The glycyrrhizic acid in licorice suggests enhanced interferon production.

Alfalfa supports central nervous system function.

Burdock cleanses liver and supports immune function.

Dandelion cleanses liver and supports health of the myelin sheath of the nerves.

Red Clover general nerve tonic.

St. John's Wort functions as an antidepressant and improves energy and appetite. New York University researchers have found the herb has dramatic action against the type of virus that causes AIDS. It contains antiviral, antibacterial, and anti-inflammatory chemicals. It is especially recommended for topical applications and internal use when cold sores are the result of a feeling of overall exhaustion. Now undergoing an FDA approval study.

Cascara Sagrada contains the active ingredient *anthraquinones* which some consider to have the ability to kill herpes simplex, reports Heniz Rosler, Ph.D., associate professor of medicinal chemistry at the University of Maryland School of Pharmacy. Use product labeled U.S.P. to make sure it has been aged for a least a year. Bark that has not been aged correctly contains chemicals that can cause violent diarrhea and severe intestinal cramps. This herb is traditionally used as a laxative and should be avoided if you are pregnant or have ulcers, ulcerative colitis, irritable bowel syndrome, hemorrhoids, or other gastrointestinal conditions.

(**Tarragon** contains caffeic acid, an ingredient that could prevent herpes as well as cancer and the flu. For a synergistic effect, drink lemon balm tea with an added teaspoon of dried tarragon. Brew for 10 to 15 minutes; drink up to 3 cups a day. Both herbs have antiviral activity.

Note: Practitioners suggest taking these herbs for short intervals, one to two weeks at a time.

Nervine and Nerve Relaxants

The central nervous system is closely related to the workings of the immune system as is the digestive system. Between them, information is constantly passed back and forth. These interdependencies of these body mechanisms are important to keep in mind when looking to heal the body of a chronic condition such as herpesvirus. Repairing the nervous system may be necessary before the immune system can be recharged.

Research shows certain herbs and grains are considered nervines or tonics for the nervous system. Common nervines include:

(Oats (tonic or in whole food form)—known for soothing the nervous and digestive systems.

(St. John's Wort—an excellent restorative for calming the

nervous system. Avoid overexposure to sunlight while taking this supplement.

- ❨ Valerian—often called the herbal Valium.
- ❨ Passion flower—soothes central nervous system.
- ❨ Skullcap—calms nervous system, cleanses liver.
- ❨ Peppermint and chamomile—are the most commonly used herbal relaxants and make soothing teas. When heated, they release compounds that have a tranquilizing effect on the body.
- ❨ Kava kava—in addition to relieving symptoms of anxiety and insomnia, it also may relieve pain and act as an antiviral and antibacterial agent.

A physician practicing in Southern California prescribes 750 mg of the amino acid GABA (gamma-aminobutyric acid) 3 times daily, after meals to calm the nerves. Magnesium (200-400 mg daily) may help balance out some of the damage caused by stress as it blocks the damaging effects of adrenaline.

Herbs for External Application

- ❨ *Aloe vera*—good overall skin healer and soother.
- ❨ *Myrrh*—in tincture form it acts as an antiseptic and anti-inflammatory effect on the mucous membranes, reduces inflammation, and speeds healing. Also contains tannins.
- ❨ *Lemon balm*—contains tannins that are useful in speeding healing and reducing pain.
- ❨ *Tannins*—while not an herb, tannins contain a variety of flavonoids and antioxidants that help heal herpes lesions. Tannins are naturally occurring substances primarily found in black and green teas, red wines, and myrrh.
- ❨ *Witch hazel*—contains compounds that show significant antiviral activity against HSV.

Red Wine Remedy

A kitchen remedy that's worth a try involves setting aside a small amount of red wine, enough to cover the bottom of the glass. Let it stand overnight. In the morning, the wine will have congealed into a concentrated form. Take a cotton swab and dab directly on sores.

Glandulars

These products act similar to homeopathic medicines as both work on the premise that like heals like. For example, taking oral glandular material of a particular animal gland will serve to strengthen the function of the corresponding human gland. The most effective are predigested soluble concentrates. Since they are predigested, the body can gain the benefits of the natural factors involved.

Thymus Extracts

Chronic infections caused by viruses, allergies, or autoimmune diseases such multiple sclerosis or lupus, often can be traced to a thymus gland functioning under par. Repetitive infections which further weaken immunity also stress thymus function.

Naturopath and author Michael T. Murray recommends a thymus extract in these situations to normalize the ratio of T-helper cells to suppressor cells and restore immune function. Since standards for glandular extracts don't exist, selecting a glandular made from a reputable manufacturer is important. According to Murray, products that are concentrated and standardized for polypeptide content are superior to crude preparations. He suggests thymus preparations contain approximately 750 mg of crude peptide fraction.

Enzymatic Therapy makes two excellent products that contain predigested thymus fractions. *ThymuPlex®* combines thymus extracts with a handful of immune-boosting antioxidants, immune-boosting herbs plus lysine. *Thymulus®* contains thymus extract with 250 mg of astragalus, which also supports immune function and boosts resistance to illness.

Homeopathy

Homeopathy can be helpful in relieving and stalling future outbreaks of herpesvirus. It is based on the theory that "like cures like" and when taken in minute doses helps the body do what it wants to do: Heal itself. It was introduced in Germany nearly 200 years ago by Samuel Hahnemann. Currently, there are more than 2,000 homeopathic preparations available, with 200 to 300 of these considered polycrest formulas, the most often used remedies.

In *The Family Homeopath* (Healing Arts Press, 1994), author Robin Hayfield concludes, "When the body becomes weakened and 'stuck' in this way, it may benefit from outside help. Homeopathy is one of the helpers. It is a way of healing that respects the body as a delicate and complete system. Used carefully, it can allow the body's own self-healing processes to work once more."

Dana Ullman, M.P.H., an author of several popular books on homeopathy, says that symptoms of illness not only represent a sign of illness, they also signify the body's best efforts to try to defend and heal itself. From this perspective, treatments such as conventional drugs that seek to stop, inhibit, or control these efforts are ignoring the body's inherent wisdom and suppressing its ability to heal itself. He also cautions that self-treatment of herpes with homeopathic medicines will commonly get rid of the eruptions quickly, but professional, constitutional care is recommended if you want to reduce the frequency or intensity of outbreaks and potentially eliminate them altogether.

In selecting a homeopathic remedy, pick the one that describes your most primary symptoms. The most often recommended homeopathic remedies for HSV-1 and HSV-2 include *Natrum muriacticum, Nitricum acidum, Sepia, Graphites, Rhus Toxicodendron,* and *Dulcamara.* For most PWH, dosages for herpesvirus eruptions are 30X potency for 2-3 days. When improvement occurs, discontinue the remedy or if there is no noticeable, positive change after 48 hours, consider trying another remedy.

For acute eruptions of herpes on the mouth: *Rhus tox* is indicated when symptoms either start at night or are worse at night and manifest as small fluid-filled blisters that itch or cause pain. *Natrum muriacticum* treats eruptions that start or are worse in the daytime and when eruptions appear at the corner or the mouth or below the corner and blisters that occur in the center of the lips. PWH who need *Hepar sulphur* have herpetic eruptions which are extremely sensitive to touch or cold.

Other effective homeopathic preparations are *Phosphorus* for cold sores that appear above the lip line and itch or cause sharp pain; *Petroleum* is indicated when sores develop loose crusts around the mouth; and *Apis* can be helpful for blisters around the lips that sting, itch, or burn. *Rhus tox* helps with fever blisters and shingles with small fluid-filled blisters that itch a lot and feel worse at night. *Graphites* is used when the blisters emit a honey-colored fluid then crust over or when there are painful cracks around the mouth. *Nitric acidum* is for blisters or ulcers on the mouth, tongue, or genitals that cause sharp pain and may bleed easily. *Dulcamara,* when aggravation is from cold, damp weather or just changes in the weather or resulting in a cold. *Capsicum* for sores that burn like hot pepper, accompanying depression or homesickness; *Tellerium* for eruptions with concurrent back or sciatica pains, and *Thuja* for people who have a history of warts, and *Sepia* for accompanying emotional distress also can be helpful.

The two most common homeopathic remedies for genital herpetic eruptions are *Natrum muriacticum* when pearl-like blisters appear and the area feels hot and swollen and *Petroleum* when symptoms are worse in the winter and better in the summer or when herpes spreads to the anus, perineum, or thighs or occurs at the onset of menstruation; when sores occur in patches, appear dark red, and are tender and moist.

For convenience, there is a combination homeopathic formula that includes some of the remedies mentioned above. *Hyland's Cold Sores and Fever Blister* combination remedy (also known as Hyland s #27) made by Standard Homeopathic is formulated to alleviate the symptoms of cold sores, fever blisters, and cracked lips from acid in food. However, you may find that an individual remedy works better, depending on your specific symptoms.

Roger Morrison, M.D., of the Hahnemann Clinic, Albany, Calif., favors homeopathy over Zorivax, the conventional prescription treatment for HSV-1 and HSV-2. He says although there are equivalent or sometimes superior responses with homeopathy without any long-term side effects, it's unclear how clinically safe the long-term use of Zorivax is.

Aromatherapy

Essential oils are at the heart of aromatherapy and have been used for hundreds of years to enhance well-being. They work on the brain, where their chemicals have an immediate effect. Joni Loughran, author, licensed cosmetologist, and consultant to several natural cosmetics manufacturers, explains in *Natural Skin Care* (Frog Ltd., 1996) that essential oils are a concentrated form of plant energy, extracted from many parts of an aromatic plant. They are much more potent than similarly dried herbs, she says.

"Aromatherapy and the use of essential oils does not cure herpes simplex 1, herpes simplex 2, or herpes zoster, but it can relieve the symptoms, reduce pain, and shorten the length of time of sores are present," says Loughran. "Because of aromatherapy's popularity, adulterated or diluted essential oils are common. When treating herpes, it's important to use high-quality, pure essential oils." (See the reference section for a list of reliable suppliers.)

According to Loughran, essential oils with antiviral properties are most helpful against herpesvirus. The ones that have shown to be safe and effective are:

- Tea tree—has antiviral, anti-inflammatory, antiseptic, and immune boosting properties. The combination of these properties makes this oil an excellent topical treatment for herpes.
- Melissa—another excellent overall oil for herpes with powerful and gentle antiviral properties. As it may cause an allergic reaction, care should be taken to apply the oil directly on the sore. Avoid surrounding tissue. While this is an expensive oil, Loughran says it is easily found in an unadulterated form.
- Eucalyptus—offers antiviral, anti-inflammatory, and antiseptic characteristics while reducing pain.

Also worth a try, says Loughran, are palmarosa and rose, as they both possess antiviral properties. She recommends combining rose with melissa. The following oils are excellent for combining with the antiviral oils mentioned above, as they reduce the discomfort associated with herpes lesions:

- Roman chamomile or German chamomile for reducing inflammation
- Bergamot (when combined with tea tree oil)

◖ Lavender for cleansing the area while reducing pain and inflammation

◖ Lemon citrus oil for its powerful antiseptic properties; also stimulates immunity. *Caution: This essential oil and sun exposure don't mix.*

Essential Oil Combinations

For cold sores, fever blisters, or facial herpes (HSV-1):

Mix together 3 drops Roman chamomile, 2 drops tea tree oil, 2 drop bergamot, and 2 drops eucalyptus. Apply to sore 3 times daily until sore begins to heal. This mixture should not be used if skin is exposed to sunlight as bergamot is photoreactive.

— or —

Combine 3 drops of tea tree oil, 3 drops melissa, and 4 drops of lavender. Apply 1 drop to sore, 3 times times daily until sore begins to heal.

◖ ◖ ◖

Each blend can be used as a compress by adding the ingredients to 2 cups cold water. Soak washcloth in mixture, wring out, and apply to affected area.

For genital herpes (HSV-2):

Mix 3 drops tea tree oil, 3 drops melissa, 3 drops Roman chamomile, and 1 drop lavender or rose oil. Add 2 tablespoons of carrier oil (canola, grapeseed, or sunflower oil). Apply to affected area 2-4 times daily.

◖ ◖ ◖

As a compress: combine 3 drops melissa, 3 drops lavender, 2 drops bergamot, and 2 drops tea tree oil with 2 cups cold water. Soak washcloth in mixture, wring out, and apply to affected area. Apply 2-4 times daily.

To maintain the integrity of these essential oil mixtures, store them in brown or dark blue glass bottles with a tight cap and place in a cool, dark place. *Discontinue use if skin becomes irritated.*

Kitchen Recipes

- Apply warm *whole* milk compresses on the lesions to help along the healing process.
- Apply a warm wet washcloth to the affected area several times a day. Follow with an ice pack made up of ice chips or cubes broken into small pieces and wrapped tightly in the center of a towel. Don't apply ice directly to lesion.
- Concentrated wine tannins. To obtain, set aside a small glass with a small amount of red wine and allow to sit overnight. Take a dampened cotton swab to transfer the dried wine to facial lesions.

Natural Products for Topical Treatment

There are several worthwhile and safe over-the-counter preparations for HSV-1 and HSV-2 available on health food and drugstore shelves. Made specifically for external application, these topical remedies for herpes blisters usually contain the healing agent allantoin, a compound from the comfrey plant, in an herbal base. Comfrey is a skin-soothing herb used in healing for more than 2,500 years.

Topicals serve two functions: To relieve pain and speed healing. Some good ones with the most natural ingredients are

Super Lysine Plus⁺ Cream™ by Quantum, Enzymatic Therapy's *Herpilyn,*™ and *Erpace*™ by Dolisos. All of these products come packaged in small tubes, making frequent applications convenient.

Super Lysine Plus⁺ Cream™ contains lysine in an olive oil base with 12 herbal ingredients, including tea tree and cajeput oils and extracts of goldenseal, echinacea flower, calendula flower, propolis plus zinc oxide, honey, gum benzoin tincture and homeopathic 3X lithium carbonate. In addition, Quantum offers two other lip preparations for cold sores and fever blisters: *LipClear*™ ointment and *LipClear Coldstick*™ containing lysine, herbs (echinacea, goldenseal, and tea tree oil), and vitamins A, D, and E in a base of a few oils. The Coldstick product also is petroleum-free, with two chemical sunscreen additives that provide SPF-15 protection. The ointment version also contains zinc oxide, a very effective sun block. Quantum topicals can be applied as often as needed. According to the manufacturer, these topicals are reported to be compatible with the company's other lysine-based supplements.

Herpilyn,™ popular in Germany before its import into the United States a few years ago, it contains a high percentage of melissa extract (lemon balm) plus allantoin. Studies have shown it very safe for adults and children, suitable for long-term use, and recommended for daily use when there are frequent recurrences of cold sores and fever blisters.

Erpace™ in addition to chamomile, oregano, and marjoram in a base of sweet almond oil, contains 1X Lappa major a homeopathic preparation, delivered by a rollerball applicator. The formula is designed to provide dry lips with moisture and to soften dry cold sores or fever blisters. It is wax- and petroleum-free. *Erpace*™ is imported from France by Dolisos.

Crystal Star also offers a line of topical remedies for various ailments including *Lysine Licorice Healing Gel.*™ It features 800 mg of lysine, licorice extract, and myrrh gum in an aloe vera base.

Less convenient but also reported effective are oils such as vitamin E, geranium, lemon, tea tree, or eucalyptus and tinctures such as myrrh. They can be applied directly to cold sores via a cotton swab every few hours. These herbs have been found to reduce pain and promote healing. However, do not apply vitamin E capsules or oil to the eye area.

There are other OTC remedies that don't meet the natural criteria but can be equally effective and sometimes are more readily available than the other preparations mentioned above. If you're traveling and can't find a store that stocks natural products, nearly every drug and mass-merchandise store in the United States stocks *Medicated Blistex®* a lip ointment, which works on cold sores and soothes dry, cracked corners of the mouth. Its main ingredient is allantoin with camphor (0.5%) and phenol (0.5%.) Camphor is considered a safe and beneficial ingredient found in skin preparations.

Whichever ready-made topical balm you apply, be sure to apply it thickly and work into the sore as much as possible, and apply at the first sign (tingling, itching, or burning) of an outbreak.

If your oral herpes is triggered by exposure to strong sunlight, there are many potent sunblocks in lip balm form. To completely block ultraviolet rays, try the bright white stuff—zinc oxide—available in drugstores or pharmacy sections of supermarkets and discount chain stores. Preparations with zinc oxide also may speed healing, as zinc oxide itself is quite drying.

What Doesn't Work

Over the years, these remedies have been tried and found ineffective and potentially harmful in relieving herpes symptoms or treating herpes lesions:

- Lasers
- Ultrasound
- Dye-light therapy with a red dye called proflavine, a light-sensitive dye that is able to penetrate the cell and the virus inside the cell. When exposed to light, the dye supposedly disrupts the viral genes so they could not reproduce and infect other cells. Once thought to be effective, it is no longer recommended for herpes treatment and is considered by many to be dangerous.
- Antibiotics—they have no effect on herpesvirus but may be used in some cases to treat secondary infections.
- Corticosteriods—creams and ointments that contain corticosteriods are used as anti-inflammatory agents. They do not seem to lessen the severity of herpes and generally are not recommended. Lesions must be kept dry with good air circulation unless they are covered by something proven to be more beneficial than dryness such as acyclovir.

Ineffective home remedies:

- Baking soda
- Peanut butter
- Watermelon
- Tea bags
- Cornstarch
- Buttermilk
- Peppermint oil
- Seaweed extracts

Ineffective store-bought remedies:

- Campho-Phenique®
- Listerine®

- Clorox®
- Spermicidal foam
- Acetone

Chapter 5

Related Conditions

Shingles

The childhood version of the herpes varicella zoster virus is known as chickenpox. Transmitted by an airborne virus, it is estimated that 75 percent of U.S. children contract the illness by age 15. If the same virus manifests itself in the same individual in adulthood, the condition is called shingles. The name comes from the Latin word *cingulus*. The *zoster* in herpes zoster takes its name from the Greek which means belt.

Shingles can reappear when the immune system is undermined by age, disease, or uncontrolled stress, and occurs most often in the elderly who often experience more severe symptoms and longer outbreaks. One estimate found that about half of people over age 80 have had shingles. It is considered a viral infection of the nerve and not a skin disease. Like HSV-1, shingles sometimes can involve the eye area, creating a condition known as herpes zoster ophthalmicus.

Shingles surfaces when herpesvirus, which has been present in the body for a long time, revives itself. Disease and uncontrolled stress also contribute to a recurrence. It gets into nerve cells, causing blisters or raised, red spots on the skin. Typically, this rash is preceded by a fever lasting 2 to 3 days accompanied by a burning irritation or sensitivity of the skin that has been compared to a severe sunburn. In about 5 days, the rash turns into blisters and then in approximately 3 days yellow lesions surface, which dry up, crust over and gradually drop off. Often a small, pitted scar is left.

Shingles appears typically on one side of the body, on the stomach under the ribs leading to the navel. Sometimes the disease affects only the lower part of the body or the upper half of the face on one side. The result is pain, itching, and burning with sores cropping up along the affected area. Even as the lesions heal, pain remains in about 5 percent of the cases. This is because the nerves have been damaged and strong impulses can remain for a long time.

The pain following an attack is a result of damaged nerves, which are passing along strong impulses to the brain. This post-shingles condition is called postviral neuralgia and affects about one-third of PWS (people with shingles). Those past age 40 are more likely to experience the post-herpetic nerve pain. The pain can be severe and last for months or even years. However, shingles is not contagious, but a person with shingles can pass on the virus, which causes chickenpox in another person.

Suggested Natural Treatments

Dietary supplements: Vitamins C and E and citrus bioflavonoids are important to effectively managing shingles. *Suggested dosages:* vitamin C: 2,000-3,000 mgs; citrus bio-flavonoids: 1g and vitamin E, 400-1,600 I.U. (taken before meals). A study conducted 50 years ago found that participants received substantial relief from intravenous doses of large amounts of vitamin C over the course of 3 to 5 days.

Vitamin B_{12}, which plays an important role in nerve function and maintaining nerve insulation (the protective myelin sheath), can not only shorten the duration of shingles but one physician believes it helps relieve pain better than anything known now. A study conducted in India found B_{12} injections relieved pain, healed blisters, and eliminated the pain associated with post-herpetic neuralgia. Injections are considered more efficient than supplements which are typically administered by physicians. *Suggested doseage:* Since B vitamins work together, take B complex (50-100 mg), 2-3 times daily and extra folic acid in addition to shots of B_{12}.

Bromelain (the active enzyme found in fresh pineapple) and pancreatin have shown to be effective anti-inflammatories. *Suggested dosages:* pancreatin: 500-1,000 mg, 3 times daily before meals; bromelain: 500 mgs, 3 times daily on an empty stomach.

Homeopathy: Ranunculus bulbous 6X, 4 times daily, then as need for pain and intense itching or when blisters are tightly grouped or appear on the trunk of the body.

Arsenicum album 30X, 2 times daily for 2-3 days at the onset and when severe burning sensation or feelings of coldness are present. Blisters typically appear clear and watery. If burning sensation persists, then switch to 12C, 2-3 times daily.

Hypericum perforatum 30X is excellent for nerve pain and symptoms of burning and tingling along the affected area. Take 2-3 times daily as needed.

Herbs: Calendula-based creams may help ease itching; and creams containing capsaicin (cayenne pepper) can help relieve pain. Zorivax and topicals containing capsaicin should be used only after all the shingle blisters have disappeared. Do not apply to active blisters.

Topical: A warm bath with a handful of cornstarch or colloidal oatmeal mixed in may soothe the skin and help with sleep. Be careful as the bottom of the tub may be slippery—be careful getting in and out of the tub.

Aromatherapy: Mix together 3 drops of Roman chamomile and 1 drop of lavender or rose. Add 2 tablespoons of carrier oil (canola, grapeseed, or safflower oil) and apply 2-4 times a day or mix 3 drops of melissa, 3 drops lavender, 2 drops bergamot, and 2 drops tea tree oil in a bowl; add 2 cups of water. Then dip washcloth in mixture, wring out, and apply to lesions 2-4 times times daily.

Also a regular practice of hatha yoga and meditation supplemented by massage is very helpful for this condition.

Prevention suggestion: Medicines containing acetaminophen are not recommended for pain relief as these OTC drugs have been found to prolong an outbreak. Also, stay away from chocolate and stressful situations as much as possible.

Canker Sores

Since they occur in the mouth, canker sores often are confused with cold sores because they also are irritating and painful. However, there are specific differences in how they appear, what causes them, and where they appear in the mouth. Cold sores appear in clusters of tiny blisters on the lips and sometimes on the gums. Conversely, canker sores tend to be smaller, crater-like lesions occurring singly or in clusters on the tongue, lips, gum, and palate as well as the lips and cheeks. Cold sores (HSV-1) are contagious; canker sores are not. An estimated 20 percent of the U.S. population is thought to get canker sores, with 10 to 40-year-olds being the age group most susceptible.

The are two kinds of canker sores, simple and complex. The simple variety last from 4 to 7 days and occur about 3 to 4 times a year. They first appear between the ages of 10 and 20, sometimes younger, but after age 21, the sores occur less frequently or stop completely. This type tends to occur in families, with more women than men affected. Complex canker sores are active in at least

50 percent of the time, resulting in a chronic condition of sores.

Causes of canker sores vary, and the biggest precipitators tend to be stress, heredity, menstruation, injury, fever, impaired immunity, or a body out of balance. Outbreaks have been noticed to be more frequent in the winter and spring than in the summer. A sensitive mouth that picks up on subtle signals of stress could also be at fault. Other researchers have found a link between hemolytic streptococcus bacteria and canker sores, with the sores a result of a hypersensitive reaction to the bacteria. Ted Grossbart, Ph.D., a Harvard Medical School psychologist, sees a specific link between emotional stress and recurrences. He has found the most common psychological triggers are stress related specifically to financial and sexual problems. Difficulty in expressing anger, he says, can also contribute to the appearance of canker sores.

Other researchers think food allergies (chocolate, nuts—particularly walnuts—and fresh citrus, particularly pineapple, and strawberries and tomatoes) also could play a role. Physical stress on mouth tissues from biting the inside of the cheek, a swipe from a hard-bristled toothbrush, or dental anesthesia canker sores. Since light and air don't easily reach the inside of the sides of the mouth, such injuries are prone to infection, and healing can be slow and often tedious process.

While doctors don't know exactly what causes canker sores, they have been found not to stem from a virus, aren't contagious, nor considered a sign of mouth cancer. A Scottish dentist, whose findings appeared in the *Journal of the American Medical Association,* concluded that patients who experienced recurrent canker sores had a singular or combined deficiency of iron, folic acid, or Vitamin B_{12}. A dermatologist with the Mayo Clinic suggests gastrointestinal diseases also can contribute to canker sores.

Other experts say that you may be able to avoid canker

sores by eating more foods rich in vitamin C, such as broccoli, cantaloupe, and red peppers. Stay away from acidic foods such as citrus fruits.

Suggested Natural Treatments

Avoid commercial toothpastes and mouthwashes. Instead use baking soda to brush your teeth and warm salt water to rinse your mouth. Then rinse with warm water with a sprinkle of dissolved sea salt, table salt, or Epsom salts. Repeat this rinse several times during the day.

To reduce pain: First, rinse your mouth with one teaspoonful of 3 percent hydrogen peroxide diluted in a small amount of water. Then take an acidophilus capsule, pierce it open, and sprinkle a small amount on the sore. Or dab a small amount of yogurt containing live cultures. Repeat every 10-15 minutes for an hour; repeat procedure in the evening. A dab of calendula or myrrh tincture applied with a cotton swab a couple of times a day should speed the healing process.

Dietary supplements: Vitamin C and B-complex.

Homeopathy: 30X, 3 times daily. *Mercurius vivus* can help at the first sign of lesions or when they appear ulcerated on the gum and tongue. *Borax* is indicated when there is a history of canker sores or concurrent hypersensitivity to noise. *Hyland's #27,* a combination remedy, may also provide relief in some cases.

Prevention suggestions: Try eating four tablespoons of unflavored yogurt daily, preferably yogurt with live cultures. (See recipe for a healthy, homemade version on page 74) The good bacterium found in yogurt are thought to stop canker sores before they develop under times of stress. Avoid coffee, spicy foods, and highly acidic foods such as tomatoes or citrus fruits.

Mouth Ulcers

Small in size, these ulcers can occur either on the tongue, gums, on the linings of the mouth or under the tongue. They typically reflect a general state of being run down, occurring most often when an individual is stressed or immunity is low. Recurring outbreaks of mouth ulcers call for longer overall treatment.

Suggested Natural Treatments

Dietary Supplements: B₂, zinc, and vitamin C.

Herbs: Myrrh in tincture form is the preferred topical remedy. It possesses both astringent and healing properties or pure wheat germ oil or vitamin E obtained by piercing a capsule containing the vitamin and dabbing some directly or on a cotton swab.

Homeopathy: 30X, 3 times daily. *Borax*—when there are small painful ulcers that feel hot in the mouth and may bleed while eating. *Mercuris Sol*—if there is metallic taste in the mouth and larger, grayish ulcers. Bleeding gums may be present. *Natrum Sulph*—for blister-like sensitive, painful ulcers. *Hyland's Formula #27,* a combination homeopathic formula also may help.

Prevention suggestion: Avoid acidic foods.

Outside the Mouth

The inflamed open cracks that appear in the corners of the mouth can often be cleared up with regular doses of vitamin B_2 (riboflavin).

Resources

BOOKS

Philosophy

Boryshenko, Joan, Ph.D. *Minding the Body, Mending the Mind.* New York: Bantam, 1988.

Carlson, Richard, Ph.D., *Don't Sweat the Small Stuff… and it's all small stuff.* New York: Hyperion Press, 1997.

Easwaran, Eknath. *Take Your Time: Finding Balance in a Hurried World,* Tomales, CA: Nilgiri Press, 1994.

_____. *Your Life is Your Message: Finding Harmony with Yourself, Others & the Earth.* Tomales, CA: Nilgiri Press, 1992.

_____. *Words to Live By: Inspirations for Everyday.* Tomales, CA: Nilgiri Press, 1996.

Elaine St. James. *Simply Your Life: 100 Ways to Slow Down and Enjoy the Things that Really Matter.* New York: Hyperion, 1994.

_____. *Inner Simplicity: 100 Ways to Regain Peace and Nourish Your Soul.* New York: Hyperion, 1995.

_____. *Living the Simple Life.* New York: Hyperion, 1996.

Homeopathy and Traditional Chinese Medicine

Kim Le, Ph.D. *The Simple Path to Health: A Guide to Oriental Nutrition and Well-Being.* Portland, OR: Rudra Press, 1996.

Pitchford, Paul. *Healing with Whole Foods: Oriental Traditions and Modern Nutrition.* Berkeley, CA: North Atlantic Books, 1993.

Cummings, Stephen, FNP, and Ullman, Dana, MPH. *Everybody's Guide to Homeopathic Medicines.* New York: G.P. Putnam's Sons, 1984.

Ullman, Dana, MPH, *The Consumer's Guide to Homeopathy.* New York: G.P. Putnam's Sons, 1995.

Diet and Recipes

Colbin, Anne Marie. *Food and Healing,* New York: Ballantine 1986.

Gittleman, Ann Louise, M.S., C.N.S. *Get the Sugar Out: 501 Simple Ways to Get the Sugar Out of Any Diet.* New York: Crown Trade Paperbacks, 1996.

_____. *Your Body Knows Best: The Revolutionary Eating Plan that Helps You Achieve Your Optimal Weight and Energy Level for Life.* New York: Pocket Books, 1997.

Krause, Pam. *Pam's Favorite Recipes* (source for sugar replacements and other sugar-free recipes). Redondo Beach, CA: Paradise Botantics Publishing, 1997. Order direct: 800/404-4770.

Turner, Kristina. *The Self-Healing Cookbook: A Macrobiotic Prime for Healing Body, Mind and Moods with Whole, Natural Foods.* Grass Valley, CA Earthtones Press, 1987.

Health and Well-Being

Hurley, Judith Benn. *Savoring the Day: Recipes and Remedies To Enhance Your Natural Rhythms.* New York: William Morrow and Co., 1997.

Huemer, Richard, M.D. and Challem, Jack. *The Natural Health Guide to Beating the Supergerms.* New York: Pocket Books 1997.

Loughran, Joni. *Natural Skin Care: Alternative and Traditional Techniques.* Berkeley, CA: Frog Ltd., 1996.

Yoga and Meditation

Easwaran, Eknath. *Meditation: A Simple Eight-Point Program for Translating Spiritual Ideas into Daily Life.* Tomales, CA: Nilgiri Press, 1978, 1991.

Farhi, Donna. *The Breathing Book: Good Health and Vitality Through Essential Breath Work.* New York: Henry Holt, 1996.

Groves, Dawn. *Yoga for Busy People.* San Rafael, CA: New World Library, 1995.

_____. *Meditation for Busy People.* San Rafael, CA: New World Library, 1993.

Lasater, Judith, Ph.D., P.T. *Relax and Renew: Restful Yoga for Stressful Times.* Berkeley, CA: Rodmell Press, 1995.
Metha, Silva, Mira and Shyam. *Yoga: The Iyengar Way.* New York: Alfred A. Knof, 1990.

Myers, Esther. *Yoga and You: Energizing and Relaxing Yoga for New and Experienced Students.* Boston: Shambhala Publications, 1997.

Pierce, Margaret D. and Martin G. *Yoga for Your Life.* Portland, OR: Rudra Press, 1996.

Zinn, Jon Kabat. *Where Ever You Go, There You Are: Mindfulness Meditation in Everyday Life.* New York: Hyperion, 1994.

ASSOCIATIONS, GROUPS, AND INFORMATION CLEARINGHOUSES

Herpes Alternative Approaches and Other Resources Page
http://users.quake.net/xdcrlab/hp/herpes/hmtl
(Can be accessed through search engines such as www.yahoo.com)

Herpes Home Page
http://www.racoon.com/newhpx.html

CDC National STD Hotline
800/227-8922   8 a.m.-11p.m. ET   M-F
Operates under a contract with the Center for Disease Control and Prevention offering information on herpes and other STDs and referrals to community support groups.

American Social Health Association (ASHA) Resource Center
(sponsored by Glaxo-Wellcome)

800/230-6039   9a.m. - 7p.m. ET   M-F
In Canada: 800/HSV-FACS
http//:sunsite.unc.edu/ASHA/

National Herpes Hotline
9 a.m - 7 p.m. M-F
919/361-8488

American Academy of Osteopathy
3500 DePauw Blvd., Suite 1080
Indianapolis, IN 46268
317/879-1881

American Association of Naturopathic Physicians
2366 Eastlake Avenue East, Suite 322
P.O. Box 20386
Seattle, WA 98102
206/323-7610

American Institute of Homeopathy
1585 Glencoe
Denver, CO 80220
303/898-5477

American Holisitic Health Association
P.O. Box 17400
Anaheim, CA 92817-7400
714/779-6152
ahha@healthy.net
Offers resources lists of professional referral organizations, plus
information research services for specific diseases and chronic
conditions. Also publishes the quarterly newsletter AhHa!.

American Holistic Medical Association
4101 Lake Boone Trail Suite 201
Raleigh, NC 27607
919/787-5181
Fax: 919/787-4916
Referrals for M.D.s and D.O.s who use complementary therapies.

American Osteopathic Association
142 E. Ontario St.
Chicago, IL 60611
312/280-5800

Center for Mind/Body Medicine
5225 Connecticut Ave. N.W. Suite 414
Washington, D.C. 20015
202/966-7338
Trains healthcare and mental healthcare professionals in
mind-body topics; also publishes a quarterly newsletter on
alternative health.

Center for Attitudinal Healing
33 Buchanan
Sausalito, CA 94965
415/331-6161
Runs support groups throughout the U.S. for people with chronic and life-threatening conditions.

American Association of Naturopathic Physicians (AANP)
2366 Eastlake Ave. E, Suite 322
Seattle, WA 98102
206/323-7610
Fax: 206/323-7612
Publishes *Journal of Naturopathic Medicine.*

National Center for Homeopathy
801 N. Fairfax St. Suite 306
Alexandria, VA 22314
703/548-7790
Provides information on homeopathic remedies; also maintains a directory of homeopathic physicians.

MAIL ORDER RESOURCES

Supplements, Herbs, and Topicals

Enzymatic Therapy
P.O. Box 22310
Green Bay, WI 54305
800/783-2286
http://www.enzy.com

Herpanacine
P.O. Box 544
Ambler, PA 19002
215/542-2981
Fax: 215/542-2983
herpana@aol.com

Hyland's/Standard Homeopathic
P.O. Box 61067
Los Angeles, CA 90061
800/624-9659
213/321-4284

East-West Herb Products
P.O. Box 1210
New York, NY 10025
800/542-6544
Bulk herbs in small quantities

Apothecarae X
1161 Cherry St. B
San Carlos, CA 94070
415/654-1795
xdcrlab@quake.net
Red marine algae, olive leaf extracts and other related products.

Hausmann's Pharmacy
534 W. Girard Ave.
Philadelphia, PA 19123

Health Concerns
8001 Capwell Dr.
Oakland, CA 94621
800/233-9355   510/639-0280
Chinese herbal preparations and books

Health Resource
1187 Coast Village Rd. Suite 1-280
Santa Barbara, CA 93108
800/366-6056
Fax: 805/965-0042
health@silcom.com

McZand Herbal
P.O. Box 5312
Santa Monica, CA 90409
Makers of the Zand line of herbal products

Nature's Herb Co.
1010 46th St.
Emeryville, CA 94608
800/365-4372

Nutrition Express
P.O. Box 4076
Torrance, CA 90510
Store location: 166 Del Amo Fashion Center, Torrance, CA
310/370-6365
800/338-7979
Fax: 310/784-8522
Discounted supplements, herbs, and personal care products

Quantum
P.O. Box 2791
Eugene, OR 94702
800/448-1448

Penn Herb Co.
603 N. Second St.
Philadelphia, PA 19123

Santa Monica Homeopathic Pharmacy
629 Broadway
Santa Monica, CA 90401
310/395-1131
Fax: 310/395-7861

Self Care Catalog
800/345-3371
SlfCare@aol.com
Herpanacine, Herpilyn, and other helpful topicals

Taos Herb Company
710 Paseo del Pueblo Sur
Cruz Alta Plaza
P.O. Box 3232
Taos, NM 87571
505/758-1991
800/353-1991
Chinese and Western herbs; supplements

United Herb Co.
P.O. Box 8005 Suite 318
Boulder, CO 80306-8005
800/864-8327
303/443-1248

Vitamin Discount Connection
645 Kolter Dr., Suite 2
Indiana, PA 15701
800/848-2990
Fax: 888/848-2329
Discounts on 400+ brands of supplements, homeopathics, books
and personal care products; also free bimonthly newsletter on
supplement research

Aromatherapy/Essential Oils

Elizabeth Van Buren Aromatherapy
800/710-7759

Essential Aromatics
800/211-1313

Original Swiss Aromatics
415/459-3998

Primavera Life in Sonoma
888/588-9830

Yoga Journal Tapes and Books
2054 University Ave. Suite 600
Berkeley, CA 94704
800/436-9642
www.yogajournal.com
Audio and video tapes on different types of hatha yoga including
Iyengar; Dr. Mary Schatz's Relaxation Tape; and nationwide
directory of yoga teachers

Iyengar Yoga Series for the Immune System with Joe Pereria
Kripa West Charity
388 Point McKay Gardens NW
Calgary, Alberta
Canada T3B 4V8
403/270-9691

Jon Kabat-Zinn's Mindfulness Meditation Practice Tapes
Stress Reduction Tapes
P.O. Box 547
Lexington, MA 02173

To order a copy of *Controlling Herpes Naturally: A Holistic Guide to Prevention and Treatment,* send your name, mailing address including zip code, and daytime telephone number to:

Southpaw Press
1653 S. 2500 E.
New Harmony, UT 84757-5083

Copies are $12.95 each plus $3 for postage and handling. Utah residents please include 6 percent sales tax. Make checks payable to Southpaw Press.

Quantities available at a discount. For information, please contact us at the above address or e-mail your request to herpesnomore@southpawpress.com.

NOTES

NOTES

NOTES

NOTES

Michele Picozzi is a health writer who specializes in natural medicine. Her articles have appeared in *Yoga Journal, New Age Journal, Delicious!, Let's Live* and *Natural Pet* as well as in medical and trade journals.